Problems and Pitfalls in Medical Literature

Adam L. Cohen

Problems and Pitfalls in Medical Literature

A Practical Guide for Clinicians

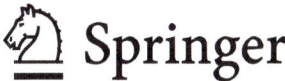 Springer

Adam L. Cohen
Medical Oncology, Internal Medicine
Inova Health System
Fairfax, VA, USA

ISBN 978-3-031-40294-4   ISBN 978-3-031-40295-1   (eBook)
https://doi.org/10.1007/978-3-031-40295-1

This Springer imprint is published by the registered company Springer Nature Switzerland AG
The registered company address is: Gewerbestrasse 11, 6330 Cham, Switzerland

Paper in this product is recyclable.

Preface

Although I have spent many years teaching medical residents and fellows about evidence-based medicine, the need for a resource on identifying problems in articles was crystallized for me at a national clinical trial meeting some years ago. A clinical trial was being proposed based on a recent article that had made a big splash in popular media after being published in a respectable medical journal. I stood up to note that the article in question had a major methodologic flaw and when that flaw was corrected, the conclusion was exactly the opposite of what the paper claimed. The speaker replied that different people had different opinions about the article. Now, there are many things one can have opinions about but statistics and methodology, in general, are not two of them. When a study is done badly, it is done badly, and no amount of hope or opinion can fix that.

This book is for medical professionals who have had some exposure to evidence-based medicine and who wish to improve their skills at reading medical literature. During medical school and residency, we pay attention to certain aspects of evidence-based medicine. We teach students to frame a question, search pubmed for articles, identify the population of an article, identify the type of article, and use statistics to calculate effects. These are important, but less attention tends to be paid to assessing the quality of an article beyond the advantages of randomization and blinding. Assessing quality is not just an essential skill for reading articles for clinical purposes. It is also an essential skill for being a peer reviewer.

Lastly, in statistics classes, much attention is paid to how to calculate various tests, like t-tests or chi-square, which many people find frightening. You will find no formulas in this book. I hope you find that fact comforting and the topic therefore less scary. When tests are discussed, it will be to note whether or not they are used properly, not to calculate them. There are statisticians with computers for a reason. This book is not for them. This book is for people who need to read medical scientific articles and decide whether what they are reading is worth remembering or not.

To approach assessing the quality of articles, some advocate a checklist approach. Checklists are useful for identifying if an article answers the question one is asking. They are less helpful for looking for fatal problems. To bowdlerize Tolstoy, good articles are all alike, but every bad article is bad in its own way. Checklists can lead to the view that one just needs enough checks to be good or that all checks are equally important, neither of which is true.

Instead, this book takes a pitfall identification view. Its goal is to give you a tool-box of the common problems and biases that are encountered in the medical litera-ture. I have divided these into categories, such as biases, which can falsely make a result tend in one direction or another; time effects, which come into play when comparing two different eras or timeframes; confounding, which occurs when an unmeasured variable affects the results; misuse of tests, which involves getting the wrong result from asking the wrong question; and power, which comes into play when studies are too big or too small. Each pitfall will be defined and an example given to illustrate how to identify the pitfall and what strategies to look for that could compensate for that pitfall. Familiarity with these pitfalls and their signs pro-vides a basis for identifying articles, often from the title, where there may be a potential problem so that you are primed to watch for pitfalls. One can then see if the authors successfully managed the potential pitfall or fell into it.

Fairfax, VA, USA   Adam L. Cohen

Contents

Part IV   Misuse of Tests

Part V   Power

Part I

Biases

Bias refers to the effects that cause an artificial deviation of a measure away from truth in a particular direction. Biases such as lead time and length time bias can affect studies of screening for disease. Immortal time bias occurs when looking at risks that take time to manifest. Ascertainment and selection bias occur when choosing patients for a study and deciding how to monitor them. Berkson's bias is a form of confounding found when selecting patients for a study who are hospitalized for unrelated diseases. Lastly, publication bias occurs when positive studies are more likely to be published than negative studies. We discuss examples of each of these biases. By understanding potential biases, the reader can identify in what direction errors may occur and see if appropriate measures to mitigate the bias have been taken.

Lead Time Bias

We have all been taught the dogma that for diseases like cancer, early detection coupled with early treatment saves lives and makes people live longer. Even for diseases other than cancer, we now recognize presymptomatic states, such as pre-diabetes or borderline hypertension, that can lead to early intervention to prevent complications. For people who have had cancer, there is high allure for tests that will both reassure that the cancer is not back but also pick it up early when it comes back, with the idea that treating it earlier will be better.

One test that at first seems to fit the bill is a blood test called CA-125 for detecting ovarian cancer. When ovarian cancer is detected at an advanced stage, it is treatable but most of the time is not cured and repeatedly recurs until the person dies from the cancer. Thus, if there were a test that could detect the cancer early, before it spreads, it could be treated with a potentially higher cure rate. Moreover, it makes sense that treating recurrences before they get too big would be more successful than treating them when they are large and causing symptoms and may have developed new mechanisms of resistance. CA-125 is a protein released from ovarian cancer cells that correlates very highly with the overall tumor mass in the body. Therefore, people have looked many times at using CA-125 to both screen for ovarian cancer and to monitor for recurrence in people who have been treated for ovarian cancer. The CA-125 is such an ingrained part of ovarian cancer monitoring that people with other cancers, like breast cancer, often ask their doctor why they aren't being monitored with such a blood test.

Lead time bias refers to the artifact of apparent improved survival when measuring survival from the time a disease is detected. Even when there is no advantage to diagnosing or detecting a disease early, people will survive longer from the time of diagnosis when a disease is detected in an earlier, asymptomatic state. The time between asymptomatic detection and symptomatic detection is called the lead time.

As an example of lead time, consider two otherwise identical women, whom we will call Alice and Betty, who both develop identical ovarian cancers at the same time in January (Fig. 1.1). For both of them, the cancer doubles in size every month, and when the cancer reaches a size that the CA-125 is above 1000, they will die of

© The Author(s), under exclusive license to Springer Nature Switzerland AG 2023
A. L. Cohen, *Problems and Pitfalls in Medical Literature*,
https://doi.org/10.1007/978-3-031-40295-1_1

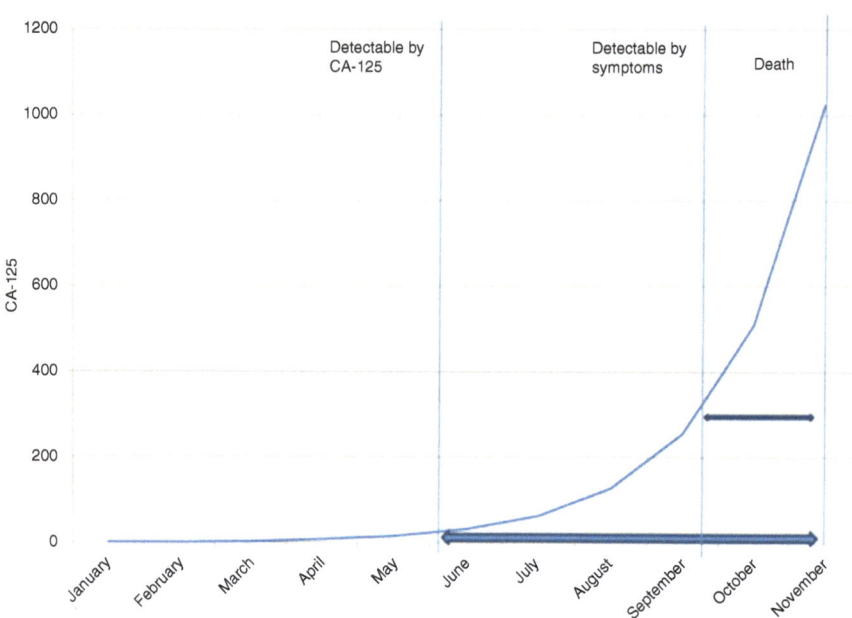

Fig. 1.1 Disease course for Alice and Betty. The thick lower arrow shows Betty's survival from the time her recurrence is found. The thinner upper arrow shows Alice's survival from the time her recurrence is found

the effects of the cancer. Alice lives a happy life for 8 months and then in October develops symptoms and is diagnosed with ovarian cancer. At that time her CA-125 is about 250. Alice has a negative attitude and does no treatment, so her cancer continues to grow, and she dies 2 months later of ovarian cancer, in December. Betty has her CA-125 drawn monthly for unknown reasons. In May, the CA-125 reaches a level where it is detectable, and Betty is diagnosed with ovarian cancer. Betty has a positive attitude and believes she can will the cancer away, so she has no other treatment. Like Alice, her cancer continues to grow at the same rate, and she also dies in December of ovarian cancer. If we were to compare how long they lived from the time of diagnosis of the cancer, it looks like Betty must have done something right, because she lived 7 months from diagnosis, while Alice only lived 2 months. That difference is misleading because in reality the difference is wehn we detected the cancer, not anything Betty did to impact the growth rate of the cancer. The 5 months that Alice knew about her cancer before Betty was the lead time. To avoid erroneously concluding that Alice's good attitude and willpower extended her life by 5 months, we need to make sure we are measuring survival from a time point that does not depend on when the cancer was detected.

Two examples of publications on ovarian cancer illustrate the dangers of lead time bias and how to avoid them. The Prostate, Lung, Colorectal, and Ovarian (PLCO) Cancer Screening Trial was one of the largest trials of cancer screening ever conducted in the United States [1]. 78,000 people, give or take, were randomized to various screening tests over an 8-year period in the late 1990s and then followed for the next 13 years. One of the interventions tested was using CA-125 blood test and transvaginal ultrasounds to screen for ovarian cancer. Half the women got the CA-125 and ultrasound and half did not. By the end of the study 212 women were diagnosed with ovarian cancer in the screening group and 176 in the control group. (See the chapter on length time bias to understand why there were more cancers found in the screening group.) People in the screening group who got ovarian cancer lived longer after the diagnosis of cancer than women in the control group, with median survival of about 5 years compared to about 3.5 years. However, when measured from the date of randomization, there was no difference in the length of survival of the women diagnosed with ovarian cancer in the two groups. In other words, women in the screening arm lived knowing they had ovarian cancer for one and a half years longer, but they died when they would have died anyway. The authors correctly identified this difference as illustrating lead time bias. In screening trials, survival or mortality should be measured from the date of randomization, not the date of diagnosis.

The MRC OV05/EORTC55955 trial examined women who had been treated for ovarian cancer and were in remission [2]. All the women saw their doctor every 3 months for a check to see if they had any symptoms of recurrent cancer. In addition, CA-125 blood tests were drawn every month. The investigators did a very clever thing, though. No one got told the results of the blood tests. The women were randomly assigned to two groups. Half the women and their doctors were told when their CA-125 level went above a predefined threshold, at which point cancer treatment was started, while half the women and their doctors were never told the CA-125 results, so they got treatment only when they started having symptoms of the cancer. Over 1400 women participated in the trial. After 6 years, the results were very clear. Both groups lived about 2 years from the time of randomization, with no difference between the groups. Cancer recurrence was detected about 5 months earlier with the CA-125 test, and those women got about 5 more months of chemotherapy, but they still died when they would have died otherwise. This is not to say the chemotherapy was ineffective. All the women got chemotherapy, and they all lived longer than they would have with no chemotherapy. It's just that the effectiveness of chemotherapy was no different based on when it was given, so any apparent benefits of treating early recurrence were based on lead time bias. Again, by looking at the survival from the time of randomization rather than from the time of recurrence detection, the authors avoided this pitfall.

References

1. Buys SS, et al. Effect of screening on ovarian cancer mortality: the Prostate, Lung, Colorectal and Ovarian (PLCO) Cancer Screening Randomized Controlled Trial. JAMA. 2011;305(22):2295–303.
2. Rustin GJ, et al. Early versus delayed treatment of relapsed ovarian cancer (MRC OV05/ EORTC 55955): a randomised trial. Lancet. 2010;376(9747):1155–63.

Length Time Bias

The goal of screening for any disease is to identify the disease in an early presymptomatic state when it can be treated or cured more easily than if it becomes symptomatic. Thus, in an ideal screening program, a simple test is done that detects an otherwise fatal or morbid disease at early stage. The medical profession then swoops in with a simple and nontoxic treatment for that early disease, curing the person who then goes on to live a long, happy life full of gratitude toward the doctors who saved their life. Everyone gets to feel good.

Lung cancer is an attractive target for screening. As the most common cancer and most common cause of cancer deaths in the United States, lung cancer is a major cause of morbidity and death. We know the major causes of lung cancer, making identification of people at higher risk easier. Lung cancers start as single tumors in the chest that grow slowly and asymptomatically for a while and can be cured with surgery if caught early enough. (Here "early enough" refers to stage 1 cancers. Lung cancers are given a stage based on how far they have spread. Stage 1 lung cancer is a single small tumor. Stage 2 is a larger tumor. Stage 3 is a tumor with cancer in regional lymph nodes. Stage 4 is cancer spread to other parts of the body that is now incurable.) Thus, the goal of lung cancer screening is to do an imaging study on asymptomatic people to find stage 1 lung cancer and perform surgery to remove the cancer. It would seem, therefore, that showing that people who have such surgery don't go on to die of lung cancer would be evidence that the screening is effective.

Length time bias refers to the tendency of screening to detect indolent disease, meaning disease that is so slow that it would not cause a problem in a person's lifetime if left untreated. It is called length time because the diseases that are around for a long time (have high length time) are more likely to be detected by screening. Imagine you have ten people with lung tumors (Fig. 2.1). Some are super-fast growing (thick arrows). These are very aggressive tumors that spend very little time as stage 1 and will become symptomatic quickly, so they will never be detected by screening. Some are medium growing (thin arrows that then become thick). These are tumors that start out slowly and spend time as stage 1 before speeding up and spreading. When these medium growing tumors are detected as stage 1 by

© The Author(s), under exclusive license to Springer Nature Switzerland AG 2023 7
A. L. Cohen, *Problems and Pitfalls in Medical Literature*,
https://doi.org/10.1007/978-3-031-40295-1_2

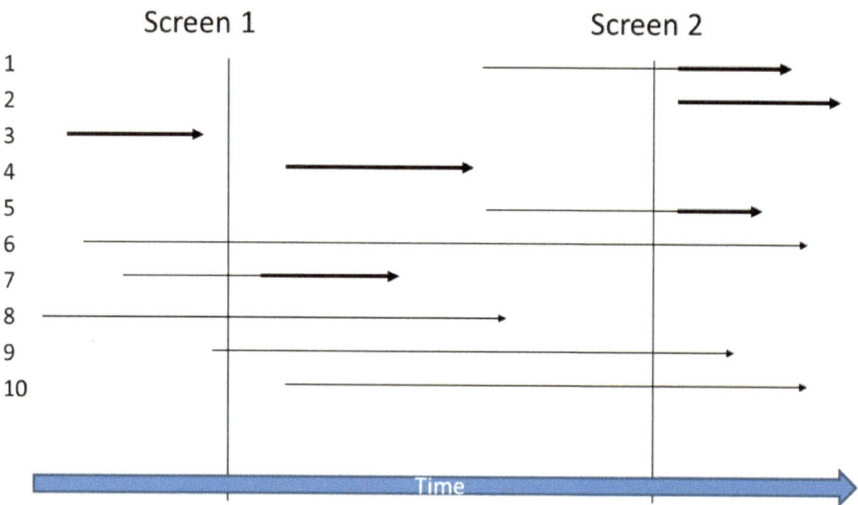

Fig. 2.1 Illustration of length time bias. More people with slower disease have disease to be found at the time of the screenings. (Figure adapted, with permission from one created by Dr. Saundra Buys)

screening, the situation is like our ideal program discussed above, where screening leads to an intervention that saves a life. These medium growing tumors are in people whose lives are saved by screening. The rest of the tumors are very slow growing (thin arrows). They stay small and stage 1 for a long time, maybe even forever. These tumors may grow so slowly that people may die of other causes without ever even knowing they had them.

In this hypothetical group of ten people, three had super-fast tumors, three had medium tumors, and four had slow tumors. However, at any given time, most of the people have slow growing tumors, because people with fast growing tumors die quickly. The vertical lines in the figure indicate two different time points when screening can occur. At the first screening time point, there are four people with tumors, of which three are slow growing (people 6, 8, and 9) and one is medium growing (person 7). At the second screening time point, there are five people with tumors, three of which are slow growing (people 6, 9, and 10) and two are medium growing (people 1 and 5). This difference in frequency of slow growing tumors, where the proportion of the screen-detected tumors that are slow growing is higher than the proportion in the general population, is length time bias.

As an example of length time bias, consider the I-ELCAP (International Early Lung Cancer Action Program) study, published in the *New England Journal of Medicine* [1]. From the title of the paper, "Survival of Patients with Stage I Lung Cancer Detected on CT Screening," we know that we are looking at how long people with early disease detected by screening are living, which is a trigger to look for length time bias and how it is handled. The paper reports the results of two rounds of screening with low-dose CT scans. The screening program detected 484 lung cancers, of which 412 (85%) were stage 1 lung cancer. This number is in stark contrast to the non-screening setting, where most lung cancers are found at later stages. In their population of people with stage 1 cancer detected by screening, 88% were still alive 10 years later, compared to 75% of people in the general population who are diagnosed with stage 1 lung cancer.

There are two possible interpretations for the data presented in the paper. The optimist interpretation is that 365 people who would otherwise have died from lung cancer had their cancer detected early and cured, i.e., they were all medium growers in our hypothetical example. The pessimist interpretation is that screening does nothing and that many of these people had tumors that would never have bothered them in their lives or were growing so slowly they would have eventually been found regardless of screening. In the pessimist interpretation, the high percentage of stage 1 tumors and the good survival of people with screen-detected stage 1 tumors are simply functions of the ability of screening to detect slow growing tumors more easily than fast ones. Because length time bias will always increase the proportion of slow growing tumors in a screened population it is impossible to tell from this paper alone without additional information that was provided by other studies which of these interpretations is true, or whether the truth is in the middle.

Reference

1. International Early Lung Cancer Action Program Investigators, et al. Survival of patients with stage I lung cancer detected on CT screening. N Engl J Med. 2006;355(17):1763–71.

Immortal Time Bias

As I was standing in my kitchen one morning making my breakfast of bran flakes and banana, my child came into the room and asked me, "Hey dad, do you know the best way to live to be one hundred?" As thoughts about non-smoking, exercise, and good genes flashed through my mind, they dead panned, "Eat an apple a day for one hundred years." This rim-shot deserving "dad joke" illustrates immortal time bias, which occurs when the exposure being measured, in this case eating apples for one hundred years, occurs over time.

Immortal time bias is also known as the Oscar bias, after the annual awards given by the Academy of Motion Picture Arts and Sciences. It is well documented that actors who win the award for Best Actor live longer, on average, than those who don't. One could imagine several reasons for this observation. For example, one could hypothesize that the gold in the Oscar statuette has properties that make the air in an actor's home healthier. Alternatively, perhaps winning an Oscar inspires actors to stop drinking, smoking, and partying and focus on their health. Perhaps one might think that some people are genetically superior with genes that both promote long life and a talent in acting. The truth is much more mundane, alas. People who die young have less chance to win an Oscar. Consider, for example, James Dean, who had acclaimed roles in *East of Eden*, released 1955, *Rebel Without a Cause*, released 1955, and *Giant*, released 1956. With the promise shown in these roles, he had the potential to win many Oscars. Unfortunately, he was killed in an automobile accident in late 1955. It would certainly be impossible for him to have an Oscar winning role after that. Contrast Dean with Henry Fonda, another iconic actor of the twentieth century. Fonda appeared in 86 movies over the course of his career, including classic performances in *Twelve Angry Men* and *Mister Roberts*, to name just two. He won the Best Actor Oscar for his performance in *On Golden Pond*, at the age of 76 years and 317 days. Less than 6 months later he died. Clearly, the Oscar statuette did not prolong his life. Rather, he happened to live long enough to be able to win an Oscar. Immortal time bias is this reversal of causation, where we think that the exposure (winning an Oscar) makes people live longer, when it is in fact the living longer that allows people to win the Oscar.

© The Author(s), under exclusive license to Springer Nature Switzerland AG 2023   11
A. L. Cohen, *Problems and Pitfalls in Medical Literature*,
https://doi.org/10.1007/978-3-031-40295-1_3

Imagine ten actors, all of whom would have the role of a lifetime that wins them an Oscar at the age of 50 (Fig. 3.1). Some, like James Dean, die young and never reach 50. Others, like Henry Fonda, may die immediately after winning their Oscar. As you can see from the figure, even with no causative relationship between winning an Oscar and lifespan, people who won the Oscar will on average live longer, because they can't win unless they have lived to be 50. The time they have to live to have the exposure is called immortal time, because the person could not have died during this time.

In medical studies, immortal time bias often shows up when looking at the relationship between side effects and efficacy. From a physiologic point of view, because both side effects and efficacy of a drug are likely related to achieving sufficient level for needed target engagement, it makes sense that people who have side effects may have greater efficacy from a drug. However, since it takes time for side effects to show up, people who have side effects will also be those who necessarily take the drug for longer. Thus, the time between when someone starts a drug and when the side effects show up is an "immortal time" that can introduce bias.

Immune therapies have revolutionized the treatment of deadly cancers like metastatic melanoma, lung cancer, or bladder cancer. Antibodies that block PD1, the programmed death protein 1, or its ligand, PDL1, activate T cells that then can attack and kill cancer cells, causing tumors to shrink and go away making people live longer. This is a good thing. Unfortunately, these T cells can sometimes get confused and attack normal tissue, causing autoimmune or immune-related side effects, such as colitis, hypothyroidism, etc. For several years, researchers have wondered if the presence of autoimmune side effects predicts benefit from immune therapy. Most studies have compared the survival of people who had autoimmune side effects with those people who don't. This situation has a great risk of immortal time bias. As my daughter would say, the best way to live a long time after being

Fig. 3.1 Illustration of immortal time among actors who would win an Oscar at age 50

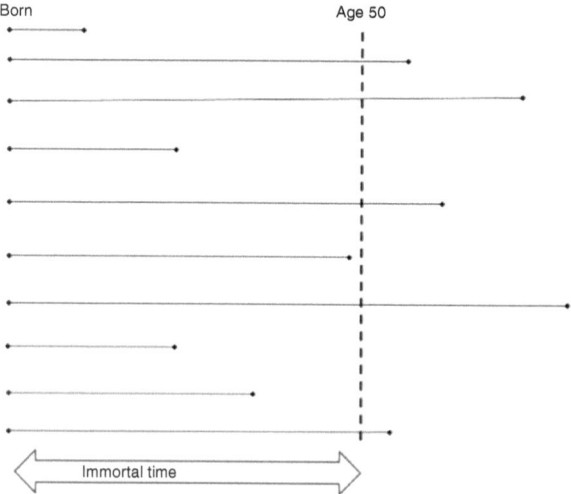

treated for bladder cancer is to live long enough to get an autoimmune side effect of your therapy.

One example of such a study was published in the prestigious *Journal of Clinical Oncology* in January 2020, by a group of authors from the FDA [1]. They examined 1747 patients from previous trials of antibodies targeting PD1/PDL1 in the treatment of bladder cancer. People who had autoimmune side effects were about three to four times as likely to see their tumors shrink after treatment (60% vs 16%) compared to people who did not have autoimmune effects. The median overall survival of people with autoimmune side effects was about 15 months compared to 6 to 7 months for those without autoimmune side effects. These results sound impressive, but do they mean that someone should worry if they don't get autoimmune side effects and feel good if they do?

One hint that the benefit seen with autoimmune side effects may be due to immortal time bias comes with looking at the timing of the side effects. In these studies 80% of the autoimmune side effects occurred after the tumor had already been shrinking from the treatment. Thus, people who had autoimmune side effects had been on treatment for a long time before the side effects came. So, did autoimmune side effects show that the treatment was working, or did people for whom the treatment was working stay on the treatment longer so that the side effects could show up?

There are several ways to try to account for immortal time bias. These authors chose to use multivariable regression where length of treatment was included as a variable. This method attempts to detect the effect of the exposure (autoimmune side effects in this case) independent of length of therapy. Although intuitively appealing, such multivariable regression is a weak way of accounting for immortal time. Because of the high correlation between length of therapy and the appearance of autoimmune side effects, the regression model can have difficulty separating their effects, leading to unpredictable results. Moreover, regression assumes a linear relationship between two variables, which may or may not be true.

Two other ways are commonly seen for dealing with immortal time bias. One good way is a landmark analysis. In a landmark analysis, one picks a time (called the landmark) after the start of the study and only looks at people who have lived at least as long as the landmark and asks the effect of having the exposure before the landmark. That's a mouthful so let's break it down using the immune therapy example. To do a landmark analysis, we would pick a time point, say 3 months after treatment starts. We would then ask, among people who have lived at least 3 months, do people who have autoimmune side effects before 3 months live longer than those who do not have autoimmune side effects before 3 months? The immortal time is eliminated because everyone in the analysis lived the 3 months and had a chance to have an autoimmune side effect during that time. Thus, landmark analyses are both simple to perform and powerful.

There are two potential downsides to a landmark analysis. The first is that the landmark time has to be chosen. Sometimes there is a logical reason to pick a landmark. For example, if one is comparing people who got 6 months of chemotherapy to people who got 12 months of chemotherapy for a cancer, it is natural to pick

12 months as the landmark time. Sometimes it is more arbitrary. The landmark time needs to be long enough to allow sufficient time for the exposure but not so long that too many people have died before the landmark is reached. The second downside is that people can continue to have events after the landmark. Thus, someone who has an autoimmune event 4 months after the start of treatment is included with people who never have an event. This misclassification may bias us toward not seeing a difference that we may have seen if we had picked a longer landmark.

The second approach for immortal time bias avoids the problem of an arbitrary landmark by allowing people to move from one group to another over time. Thus, someone who has an autoimmune event 4 months after the start of treatment would be considered to be in the no autoimmune event group for the first 4 months and in the autoimmune group after that. Such an analysis is called a time-dependent exposure or a person-year analysis. Time-dependent analyses work well when the timing of all events and potential confounders is known. In some retrospective studies, unfortunately, there is not enough data to complete a time-dependent analysis.

Once you are aware of immortal time bias, you will start to see it all over the place. Does removal of the primary tumor make women with metastatic breast cancer live longer? Does removing the ovaries of women predisposed to breast cancer reduce the risk of breast cancer? Does prescription of a statin reduce the risk of lung cancer recurrence? All of these questions are affected by immortal time bias. Anytime you can rephrase the question, "Does the occurrence of X delay the occurrence of bad thing Y?" as "The best way to avoid bad thing Y is to not have it happen long enough for X to happen"; you have the potential for immortal time bias.

Reference

1. Maher VE, et al. Analysis of the association between adverse events and outcome in patients receiving a programmed death protein 1 or programmed death ligand 1 antibody. J Clin Oncol. 2019;37(30):2730–7.

Selection Bias

4

They say the grass is always greener on the other side of the fence. In medicine, this feeling often manifests as, "Why do my patients not do as well as the patients in clinical trials?" or "Why do my patients not do as well as those reported by the big, famous academic center?" As an academic who runs clinical trials, I like to think the answer lies in the quality and structure of the care I provide. That's likely true, but the answer also lies in something just as significant. Selection bias.

Selection bias refers to the differences in outcome that result when the patients in a study are not representative of the general population. Multiple attributes can feed into selection bias, whether we are talking about a prospective study or retrospective studies. People who have good mobility will live longer than people who don't. People with normal organ function (liver, kidney, heart) will live longer than those with low organ function. People who have more indolent cancer that doesn't grow out of control while they are being screened for studies will live longer than those who don't. People who have the social and economic support to be able to travel for treatment will live longer than those who don't. People who have had fewer side effects with prior treatments and therefore feel able to do more treatment will live longer than those who don't. People who have good nutrition will live longer than those who don't. Et cetera et cetera. In short, sometimes consciously and sometimes subconsciously, researchers and clinicians tend to select for studies people who have a better prognosis, regardless of disease status, particularly when those studies involve more aggressive treatment.

Selection bias is particularly a problem for single-arm studies where a group of people are compared to "historical controls" or even contemporary controls. Indeed, when controls are contemporary, the role of selection may be even more powerful because if two people were treated at the same time but received different treatments, why was that? Even when we try to match for disease characteristics or a few other variables, it is hard if not impossible to account for everything, whether appropriate or not, that goes into clinical discussions and decisions.

One of the longest and saddest examples of the impact of selection bias comes in the treatment of breast cancer with high-dose chemotherapy with autologous stem

© The Author(s), under exclusive license to Springer Nature Switzerland AG 2023
A. L. Cohen, *Problems and Pitfalls in Medical Literature*,
https://doi.org/10.1007/978-3-031-40295-1_4

cell rescue, otherwise known as bone marrow transplants for breast cancer. In the 1980s, chemotherapy was shown in randomized trials to be beneficial in both early and late breast cancer. Given those results, it was natural to ask: "If some chemotherapy is good, is more better?" Unsurprisingly, in the late 1980s and early 1990s reports began to be published of single-institution series of treating women with late-stage breast cancer with high-dose chemotherapy with good results. Women treated with high-dose chemotherapy had long-term cancer control and lived longer than would have been expected, leading to great enthusiasm. High-dose chemotherapy became the rage and women and activists demanded access to this seemingly life-saving therapy. (For a detailed discussion of the history of high-dose chemotherapy in breast cancer, read the highly readable *Emperor of All Maladies* by Siddartha Mukherjee.) Eventually, randomized trials and evidence-based reviews showed that there was no benefit to high-dose chemotherapy. It was all selection bias. (Actually, not all, there was some fraud too, but that's a different story.) So what happened?

It starts with small, single-institution studies. For example, in 1988, the *Journal of Clinical Oncology* published a phase II, single-arm, single-institution trial of high-dose chemotherapy as first-line treatment for women with metastatic breast cancer. (This paper was neither the first nor any different in quality than others, but we have to pick one to look at.) In it, 22 women were treated. The complete response rate was 54%, which is incredibly high. For women who achieved a complete response after 18 months of follow-up most of the women were still alive, which again was impressive. Thus, although 5 of the women died from toxic side effects of the treatment, further study was felt to be indicated. Note that the average age of women in this study was 36, with none over the age of 50, and all had normal heart, liver, and kidney function [1].

By the end of the 1990s thousands of women had been treated with high-dose chemotherapy. In 1999, *JAMA* reported the outcomes from 1188 women in the Autologous Blood and Bone Marrow Registry. In their multivariate analysis, time to treatment failure after high-dose chemotherapy was better for women under the age of 45, with high performance status (Karnofsky score 90 or 100), who had never received chemotherapy before, had no cancer in their liver or brain and had only 1–2 sites of chemotherapy, and whose tumors shrank in response to chemotherapy before the high-dose chemotherapy. There are two ways to interpret such differences. One is to say that people who don't meet these criteria should not receive high-dose chemotherapy and that women who do meet these criteria should. Another is to wonder whether these women would do just as well no matter what they got [2].

In fact, as randomized trials would later confirm, this answer was already known. In 1997, *the Journal of Clinical Oncology* published two articles aptly named "Patient Selection in High-Dose Chemotherapy Trials: Relevance in High-Risk Breast Cancer" and "Impact of Selection Process on Response Rate and Long-term Survival of Potential High-Dose Chemotherapy Candidates Treated with Standard-dose Doxorubicin-Containing Chemotherapy in Women with Metastatic Breast Cancer" [3, 4]. Both articles showed the same thing, namely that women who met all the criteria for high-dose chemotherapy (young, otherwise healthy, good

**Table 2. Selection Criteria for HDCT and Number
of Patients Excluded by Each Criterion**

Eligibility Criterion	No. of Patients Excluded (%)*
CR or PR to doxorubicin-based SDCT	552 (34.9)
Age = 60 years	444 (28)
PS ≤ 2 (Zubrad)	211 (13)
Bilirubin ≤ 2 mg /dL	28 (2)
Platelets ≥ 100,000/μL	22 (1.4)
Symptomatic cardiac dysfunction	5 (0.3)
WBC count ≥ 2,000/μL	3 (0.2)
All criteria combined	936 (59)

Abbreviations: PR, partial response; CR, complete response.
*The number of patients excluded by each criterion alone from the total
of 1,581 patients.

Fig. 4.1 Effect of various inclusion criteria on eligibility for treatment. (Reprinted with permission from Rahman et al., "Impact of selection process on response rate and long-term survival of potential high-dose chemotherapy candidates treated with standard-dose doxorubicin-containing chemotherapy in patients with metastatic breast cancer", Journal of Clinical Oncology vol 15, no. 10 (October 01, 1997) 3171–7. https://ascopubs.org/doi/pdf/10.1200/JCO.1997.15.10.3171 ?role=tab)

performance status) lived significantly longer than women who don't meet those criteria even when treated with standard-dose chemotherapy and that when one looked at these young, healthy women and compared those who had received standard chemotherapy with those who received high-dose chemotherapy, survival did not differ (Figs. 4.1 and 4.2).

Despite all we have learned in the subsequent years, selection bias continued to rear its ugly head in the medical literature. Why? It takes a lot of resources to do large, multicenter, randomized trials with representative populations. This resource barrier leads to two implications. The first is that it is cheaper, faster, and easier to report on a small group of selected patients, and journals want to publish exciting, promising results. The second is that to justify a large, expensive trial, preliminary data is needed, and where does preliminary data come from? Small, single-center studies with historical controls.

As the above examples illustrate, there are several signs to look for to identify selection bias that could be making results look better than they truly are:

- Unusually young population
- A treatment that only particularly healthy people can tolerate, like organ transplantation
- A treatment that takes a long time to prepare, so people with faster grower disease won't make it to treatment
- Treatment that people with only a small volume of disease are eligible for
- Treatment that people have to travel to a specialized center for
- Small group enrolled over a long period of time
- Population restricted to one ethnic group or gender without reason

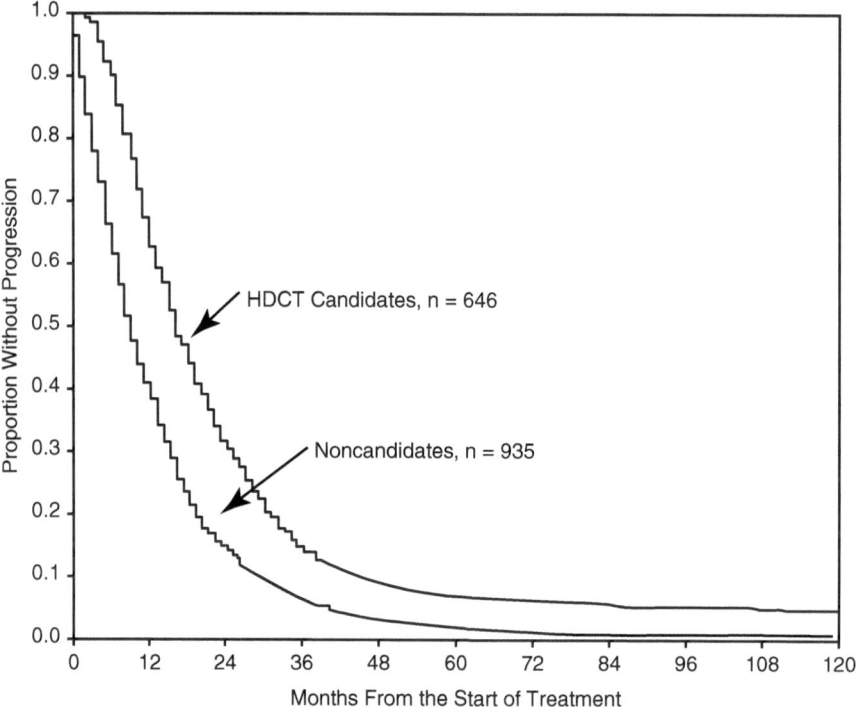

Fig. 4.2 Impact of selection criteria on survival, despite similar treatment. (Reprinted with permission from Rahman et al., "Impact of selection process on response rate and long-term survival of potential high-dose chemotherapy candidates treated with standard-dose doxorubicin-containing chemotherapy in patients with metastatic breast cancer", Journal of Clinical Oncology vol 15, no. 10 (October 01, 1997) 3171–7. https://ascopubs.org/doi/pdf/10.1200/JCO.1997.15.1 0.3171?role=tab)

Therefore, when you see a headline like "Selected Patients with Nonresectable Colorectal Liver Metastases had long survival after liver transplant with survival exceeding that of patients treated with portal vein embolization," you should think, "Of course, selected patients did."

References

1. Peters WP, et al. High-dose combination alkylating agents with bone marrow support as initial treatment for metastatic breast cancer. J Clin Oncol. 1988;6(9):1368–76.
2. Rowlings PA, et al. Factors correlated with progression-free survival after high-dose chemotherapy and hematopoietic stem cell transplantation for metastatic breast cancer. JAMA. 1999;282(14):1335–43.
3. Garcia-Carbonero R, et al. Patient selection in high-dose chemotherapy trials: relevance in high-risk breast cancer. J Clin Oncol. 1997;15(10):3178–84.
4. Rahman ZU, et al. Impact of selection process on response rate and long-term survival of potential high-dose chemotherapy candidates treated with standard-dose doxorubicin-containing chemotherapy in patients with metastatic breast cancer. J Clin Oncol. 1997;15(10):3171–7.

Ascertainment Bias

5

Among the more confusing statistical terms is ascertainment bias. The word ascertainment means the process by which something is found out. The confusion stems, in part, from the fact that the term ascertainment bias can mean several different things based on what the "something" being found out is. Some situations of ascertainment bias overlap with other biases we discuss, like confounding (discussed later) or selection bias. Although academic arguments about exactly which term to use in any given situation have their role, for the consumer of medical literature such arguments are beside the point. No matter what you call something, the goal remains to identify the presence of a bias, what the potential effect of that bias is, and how to mitigate it. We will look at ascertainment bias in two contexts.

The first context for ascertainment bias is genetic studies. In some ways, studies of genetic predispositions to a disease are models for any study trying to determine how likely an outcome is based on some risk factor. In genetic studies, the "something" being found out is typically people or families with a genetic risk factor for a disease. What patients and providers want to know is: if a person has a pathogenic gene, what is the chance of developing the disease by a certain age? To calculate this chance, we need a bunch of people with the gene and then we need to see how many of them develop the disease at each age. The bias comes in when we collect the people with the gene. How we ascertain who has the gene will affect the chance of developing the disease we calculate at the end.

When a gene (or other cause of a disease) is first discovered it will be in a group with a high likelihood of that disease. For genetic studies, this means families with a lot of people with that disease. If you are going to look for a gene that causes breast cancer, start in a family with lots of breast cancer. These families with a high level of a disease may have multiple factors contributing, however. Thus, due to how we ascertain these first cases, initial estimates of how risky a particular gene (or other risk factor) is tend to be overestimates. As we look more widely, we will discover families with the same gene but lower risk.

As an example, consider the BRCA1 gene, which predisposes to breast and ovarian cancer. BRCA1 was discovered as a risk factor for breast cancer in the 1990s. It

© The Author(s), under exclusive license to Springer Nature Switzerland AG 2023

A. L. Cohen, *Problems and Pitfalls in Medical Literature*,

https://doi.org/10.1007/978-3-031-40295-1_5

got a lot of popular attention in 2013 when the actress Angelina Jolie wrote a *New York Times* column about her experience as a carrier of a pathogenic variant in BRCA1. As she wrote, "My doctors estimated that I had an 87% risk of breast cancer." Is that right? It turns out that 87% was the initial estimate of lifetime risk of breast cancer in the families where BRCA1 was discovered. Figure 5.1, which I estimated based on a combined analysis of retrospective studies through 2003, shows how the estimate of risk of breast cancer in BRCA1 varied over the years based on the year of publication [1]. Although the initial estimates were as high as 90% risk of breast cancer by age 80, over time it became clear that many people with BRCA1 pathogenic variants have a much lower risk of breast cancer, which can be better estimated by knowing what mutation they have and what their family history is. More recent, prospective studies have shown that in the whole population of people with BRCA1 pathogenic variants, the rate is probably about 40–50% with the individual risk influenced by the family history. The ascertainment bias of looking initially in families with high rates of breast cancer caused an overestimation of risk for other families with BRCA1 who may have differed from the original very high-risk families based on other genetics or environment.

The second context where ascertainment bias can be seen is when there is different monitoring between groups. In general, when someone is sick, healthcare interventions are a good thing. Even when one can't help the underlying disease, paying close attention to someone can help them get better faster. Whether it is a form of placebo effect or whether close monitoring allows small problems to not develop into big problems is not important. The important point is that people who are monitored more closely do better.

The impact of monitoring was illustrated by a classic paper by Antman et al. on a clinical trial on sarcomas [2]. They looked at a clinical trial of chemotherapy after resection of soft tissue sarcomas. Ninety people were considered eligible for the trial. Of these, 52 enrolled on the trial, 24 had physicians who chose not to enroll them on the trial, and 24 refused to enroll on the trial. The 52 people enrolled on the trial were randomized to receive chemotherapy or observation. Of the people not on the trial, some people chose to receive chemotherapy and some chose not to. Thus, there are four groups of people, those who received chemotherapy as part of the trial, those who received chemotherapy not as part of the trial, those who were

Fig. 5.1 Relationship between year of publication and estimated risk of cancer in BRCA pathogenic variant carriers by age 50 and 80

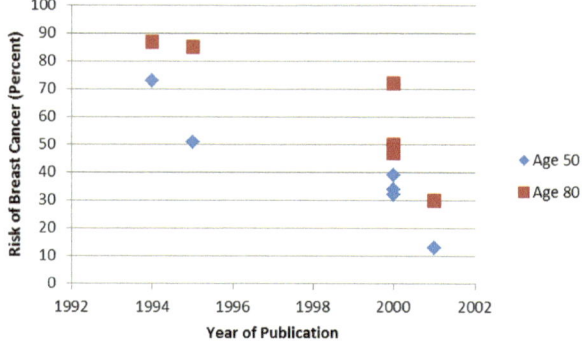

observed as part of the trial, and those who were observed not as part of the trial. Two years after surgery, 50% of people who were observed not as part of the trial were alive without cancer recurrence, 65% of people who were observed as part of the trial were alive without cancer recurrence, 70% of people who received chemotherapy not as part of the trial were alive without cancer recurrence, and 80% of people who received chemotherapy as part of the trial were alive without cancer recurrence. This survival benefit of being in the trial is partly due to selection bias and partly due to ascertainment, namely that people in the trial are monitored closely which improves their outcomes.

Fortunately, very obvious ascertainment bias, such as one group being monitored every 5 months and another group being monitored every 2 months, is rare. It is important to be mindful for differences in how often people are monitored or seen because even subtle differences can sometimes make big differences.

References

1. Antoniou A, et al. Average risks of breast and ovarian cancer associated with BRCA1 or BRCA2 mutations detected in case series unselected for family history: a combined analysis of 22 studies. Am J Hum Genet. 2003;72(5):1117–30.
2. Antman K, et al. Selection bias in clinical trials. J Clin Oncol. 1985;3(8):1142–7.

Publication Bias

6

Not everything in medicine gets reported. There are multiple reasons some cases and some trials get published and others don't. Negative results are less likely to be reported than positive results. This deficiency results both from self-censoring and from editorial bias. Consider two scenarios. Dr. A has a patient with a rare metastatic toenail cancer. She sequences the tumor and finds a mutation in the KRAS oncogene. Although there are no publications on KRAS inhibitors in metastatic toenail cancer, she gives the patient a KRAS inhibitor and the tumor shrinks away. Based on these good results, she writes a case report describing the first successful use of a KRAS inhibitor in metastatic toenail cancer, and it is published in a prestigious journal. Dr. B has a patient with a rare metastatic fingernail cancer. He sequences the tumor and finds a mutation in KRAS. Although there are no publications on KRAS inhibitors in metastatic fingernail cancer, he gives the patient a KRAS inhibitor. Unfortunately, the tumor continues to grow quickly and the patient dies 6 weeks later. Dr. B is busy and not excited about writing a report that he worries will make him look bad. Eventually, he gets around to writing a case report and submits it to a journal, but it is rejected because the reviewer had many questions about the dose used and whether the results have an impact on the field.

As these examples illustrate, the published literature is going to be weighted toward reports that are positive with an underrepresentation of negative results. Although it is easy to see how this discrepancy could happen with case reports, such publication bias can also happen with large prospective trials. Both because of self-censoring due to time constraints and self-interested delays in publishing negative results, negative results take longer to publish after studies end and are more likely to never be published. Of phase II and phase III trials in breast cancer, fewer than half are published within 5 years, even when results have been presented at meetings. Moreover, positive studies are six times more likely to be published than negative studies [1]. Similar results have been seen in other diseases.

As an example, consider the case of erythropoiesis-stimulating agents (ESAs) in cancer. ESAs boost red blood cell production, decreasing the level of anemia that can occur due to cancer or to treatments of cancer. The theory was that by

A. L. Cohen, *Problems and Pitfalls in Medical Literature*,
https://doi.org/10.1007/978-3-031-40295-1_6

23

decreasing anemia, people would have more energy and feel better. In 2014, Bohlius et al. published in the *British Journal of Cancer* a meta-analysis of all the prospective randomized clinical trials they could find on the effects of ESAs in people with cancer [2]. They examined 37 randomized clinical trials of EPAs with quality of life data. Of these, they were able to include 7 that had not been fully published. Thus, at least 20% of the trials would have been missed if they had looked only at published papers. Overall they concluded that ESAs had a clinically insignificant effect on fatigue (measured by a scale called FACT-F) and a barely clinically significant effect on anemia-related symptoms (measured by a scale called FACT-An).

To examine the role of publication bias, one common method is called a funnel plot. The following discussion gets a bit heavy into these graphs. The important thing to know is that a meta-analysis or systematic review should include a funnel plot and make a statement about whether publication bias is likely present or not. If you don't see one, you should worry. If you don't care about reading a funnel plot, skip to the last paragraph in this section.

In a funnel plot, each study is plotted on a graph (Fig. 6.1). The x-axis is the effect size measured in that study. For the ESA studies, that would be the difference between the groups (those who used ESAs and those who did not) on the quality of life scales, FACT-F or FACT-An. The y-axis is a measure of the size of the study. Sometimes the y-axis will be the actual sample size. Sometimes it will be the standard deviation or standard error of the measure used for the x-axis. Recall that sample size and standard error are related, such that the larger the sample size the smaller the standard error and vice versa. So, in the funnel plots from the ESA analysis, the top of the y-axis, where standard error is smallest, is where the larger studies are, and the bottom of the y-axis, where the standard error is smallest, is where the smaller studies are. In general, we expect larger studies to be more accurate and to have an effect size close to the true value, while smaller studies will have a larger range of effect sizes whose average is still the true value. Thus, the graph should look like a funnel with points tightly clustered at the top and then fanning out the lower on the graph you look. A line is drawn estimating the relationship between the effect size and the study size, which should ideally be a vertical line at the average effect size, which is the best estimate of the true effect. Error bars around this line should be wide at the bottom and narrow at the top, like a funnel. The points that represent the studies should be symmetric around the line representing the average effect/true effect, because we expect that randomly about half of studies will overestimate the true effect and half will underestimate it.

Looking at the funnel plots from the ESA studies, first look at graph B, which is for the FACT-An scale. It looks similar to what a funnel plot should look like. The solid line with the average estimate is vertical. The points are roughly symmetric. There probably should be a couple of small studies with larger effect sizes, but the p-value tells us that differences from a symmetric funnel can be random. (Egger's test is a way to measure whether the funnel plot deviates from the expected funnel. You don't need to worry about how to calculate Egger's test or what it is, unless you want to do a meta-analysis. For reading meta-analysis, all you have to know is that if the Egger's test is significant, then that suggests publication bias may be present.)

Fig. 6.1 Funnel plot examples. (Reprinted with permission from Bohlius J, Tonia T, Nuesch E, Juni P, Fey MF, Egger M, et al. Effects of erythropoiesis-stimulating agents on fatigue- and anaemia-related symptoms in cancer patients: systematic review and meta-analyses of published and unpublished data. Br J Cancer. 2014;111(1):33–45)

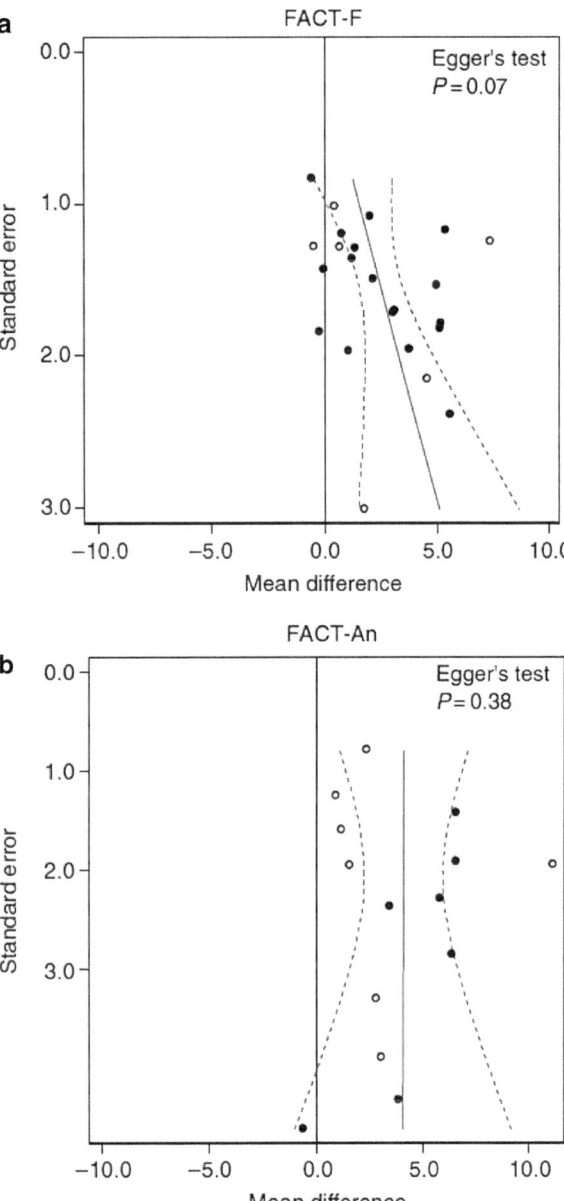

Note that in the FACT-An graph, the open circles are from unpublished reports. Note how the effect size (mean difference on the x-axis) is larger in the published reports, represented by closed circles, so if only the published reports had been included, the effect size would have been overestimated due to publication bias.

Now look at the graph A, which shows the funnel plot for the FACT-F scale. Here there is more reason for concern. Visually, we see that the solid line is not straight, meaning the estimate from small studies is different than large studies. The Egger's test *p*-value is borderline at 0.07, suggesting there may be asymmetry and that there may be other unpublished studies found. Again, also note that the large unpublished studies tended to have smaller effect sizes than other studies. The funnel plot doesn't say that the FACT-F results are invalid, just that we should think about them more deeply and consider them potentially less accurate than other results.

The requirement to pre-register clinical trials helps with understanding the prevalence of publication bias. All clinical trials are required by both regulations and rules of the International Committee of Medical Journal Editors to register before they start. There are some international databases, but the most commonly used database for registering is www.clinicaltrials.gov, which is an excellent resource for identifying clinical trials that have been done.

References

1. Song SY, et al. The significance of the trial outcome was associated with publication rate and time to publication. J Clin Epidemiol. 2017;84:78–84.
2. Bohlius J, et al. Effects of erythropoiesis-stimulating agents on fatigue- and anaemia-related symptoms in cancer patients: systematic review and meta-analyses of published and unpublished data. Br J Cancer. 2014;111(1):33–45.

Berkson's Bias

7

People who interact with the healthcare system tend to be sick, which may seem obvious. One explanation is that some people who are healthy and never injure themselves never have reason to be admitted to a hospital. However, the relationship between interactions with the healthcare system and sickness go deeper. Don't worry, this is not a conspiratorial screed about how hospitals actually make people sicker. No actual people were harmed in the making of this chapter. Instead, we will look at how the mere act of hospitalization affects the apparent associations of disease.

First, let me convince you that there is a problem. The problem goes by several names, including Berkson's bias, admission bias, or informed presence bias. In 1946, Berkson was examining whether gall bladder disease caused diabetes. (Short answer, it doesn't, though given their anatomic proximity it was a reasonable hypothesis at the time.) He did a case-control study in a group of hospitalized people comparing the rate of gall bladder disease in those with diabetes and those without. He found a statistical association of the two diseases. However, he then looked at the same two diseases in the general population and found no association. Thus, by studying a hospitalized population one would erroneously conclude that gall bladder disease causes diabetes when it does not.

There are several reasons that people who are admitted to a hospital or interact a lot with the medical system are more likely to show erroneous associations between diseases. These reasons are confounding variables, meaning they correlate with both variables one is looking at, in this case diabetes and gall bladder disease. Confounders are one of the things that make "correlation is not causation" the mantra of statistics students everywhere. First, people who have more diseases are more likely to be hospitalized because they tend to have more complications from a disease. Thus, if two people show up with gall bladder disease but one has diabetes and the other does not, the one with diabetes is more likely to be hospitalized because they are more likely to have more complicated gall bladder disease. This tendency leads to any two diseases being associated in a hospitalized population. Second, people who are hospitalized or who have a lot of contact with the medical system

© The Author(s), under exclusive license to Springer Nature Switzerland AG 2023
A. L. Cohen, *Problems and Pitfalls in Medical Literature*,
https://doi.org/10.1007/978-3-031-40295-1_7

tend to pick up diagnoses, particularly for things with minimal symptoms. Thus, if someone has early diabetes they may get diagnosed with it when they are hospitalized for gall bladder disease and their labs happen to show diabetes. Third, the presence of other conditions that lead to multiple diseases, such as immobility, smoking, or obesity, is more common in hospitalized populations, so associations may be seen due to the presence of a common risk factor. These conditions are confounding because they can cause both diabetes and gall bladder disease, which makes it appear there is a correlation of diabetes and gall bladder disease even though one does not cause the other. For these reasons, examining case-control or cohort studies in people who are hospitalized or have many contacts with the medical system can lead to spurious associations.

As an aside, there is also a way that one can see a spurious negative association by looking in hospitalized populations if the copresence of disease does not increase the risk of hospitalization. Suppose you are looking at the relationship of gall bladder disease and diabetes and it turns out that having one has no impact on the chance of getting hospitalized (note the word hospitalized not occurrence) of the other. To be simple, let's also assume the hospital is full of people who were admitted either for gall bladder disease or diabetes. In that case, everyone who was admitted without having diabetes must have gall bladder disease and vice versa. We would then see a spurious negative association between the two, because we have weeded out a large population of people who have neither of them.

As the density of the above paragraphs indicates, identifying Berkson's bias can be tricky and subtle at times as is figuring out how it affects data. Particularly in the modern world of big data and large electronic medical records, it is tempting to think that size and statistical adjustment for confounders can solve all problems. It is sobering and humbling to remember that we have to think about the effects of where the data we use comes from.

As an example, consider the research on whether monoclonal gammopathy of uncertain significance (MGUS) leads to deep vein thrombosis (DVT). MGUS is a precursor condition to the cancer multiple myeloma. It is well described that, like many cancers, multiple myeloma increases the risk of blood clots such as DVT. It has been an open question whether the precursor MGUS did the same thing. The important thing to know about MGUS is that it is, by definition, asymptomatic. It is a pure lab test abnormality that is found when investigating some other problem. Thus, people with MGUS will either have other medical problems, such as kidney disease or neuropathy, that led to their being checked for MGUS, or they will see a doctor and have enough blood tests for someone to notice high protein levels, which can be an indicator of MGUS.

In 2008, Kristinsson published a large study looking at the relationship between DVT and MGUS [1]. They included over four million US veterans who had been hospitalized at a VA hospital. (Note the two tip-offs to potential Berkson's bias: the use of hospitalized patients and a disease that only shows up in the workup of other diseases.) They found an incidence of DVT in people with MGUS of 3.1/1000 person-years compared to 0.9/1000 person-years in people without MGUS, which is a relative risk of 3.3. The relative risk was even higher in the first year after

MGUS diagnosis at 8.6. (This higher risk in the first year is another tip-off that something statistically amiss may be going on. If MGUS is doing something biologic, that biologic risk for DVT should remain stable or increase the longer one has MGUS. On the other hand, if the diagnosis of MGUS and diagnosis of DVT are being associated because of something else that leads to hospitalization, then you would expect a big DVT risk around the time of MGUS diagnosis but not at other times.)

There are a number of ways to deal with Berkson's bias. One is to not limit your population to hospitalized patients and to look in the general population. Another is to look at other random diseases to see if they are also correlating with your disease of interest. A third is to control for contact with the healthcare system, such as by adjusting for number of hospitalizations or number of clinic visits or number of other diagnoses.

In looking at the relationship of DVT and MGUS, different groups have used many of the above techniques. For example, one group compared the DVT rate in veterans with MGUS to the DVT rate in veterans who had been tested for MGUS and found not to have it. Because MGUS is asymptomatic, using this control group allowed the inclusion of a group that was similarly sick and had similar other risk factors to the MGUS group. Because this control group had a higher rate of DVT than the general population, the relative risk for DVT in the MGUS population was decreased to a nonsignificant 1.38, indicating that the apparent association of DVT and MGUS was not due to a strong biologic effect but rather to a form of Berkson's bias in which people who are hospitalized for diseases associated with DVT risk are also at risk for being diagnosed with MGUS.

Reference

1. Kristinsson SY, et al. Deep vein thrombosis after monoclonal gammopathy of undetermined significance and multiple myeloma. Blood. 2008;112(9):3582–6.

Part II

Time Effects

Time effects occur when the passage of time becomes a confounding factor in study results. The Hawthorne effect refers to how people change behavior when they know they are being observed. In medical studies, the Hawthorne effect often comes into play when a study looks at outcomes before and after some intervention. The Will Rogers effect refers to how a measure can improve in two subgroups when recategorizing people from one subgroup to the other, even when the measure has not changed for any individual person. We see this effect in medical studies when diagnostic criteria change over time, often referred to as stage migration or cohort effects, making people in one time period not comparable to people in another time period. We look at examples of both the Hawthorne effect and the Will Rogers effect in recent articles.

Hawthorne Effect

8

It may be hard to believe, but people behave differently in public and private. When people know they are being watched, they do things they might not otherwise do, at least until they get tired of it, and they don't do things they might otherwise do, like pick their nose. People also like being cared about. When a group of people knows their leaders are interested in them, they will work harder or better, at least temporarily. These seemingly self-evident truths are the basis of the Hawthorne Effect.

The Hawthorne Effect is named after the Hawthorne Works, which was a factory outside of Chicago that made electrical supplies. In the late 1920s and early 1930s, the leaders of the Hawthorne Works wanted to increase production, so they talked to experts and did a series of studies on changing conditions at the factory. No matter what they did, it always seemed to increase production for a few weeks and then production would go back to normal. When they turned the lights up to make the factory brighter and more cheerful, production went up temporarily. When they turned the lights back down so workers wouldn't be distracted, production went up temporarily. A later researcher, Henry Landsberger, first used the term Hawthorne Effect to describe improved performance during an intervention because subjects know they are being observed. It is the act of observing that changes behavior, not the intervention itself. In the medical literature, the subjects may be patients or they may be staff, depending on the particulars of the study.

Given its origins, the Hawthorne effect is easiest to see in quality improvement studies that employ a before-and-after design where a quality outcome is measured after a new intervention and then compared to that same measure before the intervention. For example, while receiving courses of radiation treatment, patients should be seen by the radiation doctor about once a week to assess for side effects in what is called an on-treatment visit (OTV). One radiation oncology department at a safety-net hospital recognized that patients were not realizing they need to go to the OTVs despite verbal reminders from the technicians. They implemented a plan in which brightly colored paper was given to the patients as a reminder with the idea that if the patients did not head toward the OTV area of the clinic, staff would see the bright paper and redirect them. Quite clever really. They looked at how many

A. L. Cohen, *Problems and Pitfalls in Medical Literature*,
https://doi.org/10.1007/978-3-031-40295-1_8

OTV visits were missed in the year before the bright paper intervention and during the year after the bright paper intervention [1]. Before the intervention, 7.7% of OTVs were missed vs 1.3% in the year after the intervention, which was statistically significant with $p = 0.007$. They conclude that, "This simple, inexpensive intervention that circumvents cultural, language, and medical literacy barriers may be easily implemented throughout radiation oncology practices to improve patient care."

We all want to believe that we have control over our behavior and that what we do matters for the reasons we think it does. It is possible that the bright paper was necessary and sufficient to lead to long-term behavior change. It is also possible that any intervention would have had a similar effect because the staff knew OTVs were a priority during this time and knew OTVs were being measured, leading to a Hawthorne Effect. Mitigating the Hawthorne effect could be done in a couple of different ways. One is to use a parallel or randomized design rather than a before-and-after design, so that the control group is measured at the same time as the intervention group, which reduces the effect of other behavior changes the staff might be undergoing. The second way is to have some minimal intervention for the control group so that the attention and knowledge about observation is similar before and after the current intervention.

The Hawthorne effect can affect studies of patients in addition to quality studies of providers. In some ways, the Hawthorne effect is like the placebo effect, except that instead of people getting better because they think they are getting medicine, people get better because they are being watched and feel cared for. Consider the SymptomCare@Home study [2]. In this randomized study, people beginning chemotherapy for cancer were randomized to usual care or to an intervention in which they reported daily symptoms via telephone, and if the symptom level was high enough they got a call from a nurse practitioner to discuss their symptoms. Neuropathy is one dreaded side effect of chemotherapy that can cause numbness, tingling, or burning pain in the extremities due to damage to long nerves in the body. The important thing to know about neuropathy is that there are no proven treatments for neuropathy that have any but a small effect, except by changing the cause of the neuropathy. Nonetheless, the patients in the intervention group had significantly fewer days with moderate (1.8 days vs 8.6 days) or severe (0.3 days vs 1.1 days) neuropathy symptoms, despite no change in the underlying cause, which is the chemotherapy. We know from other randomized trials that no drug or behavior intervention has such a large effect on neuropathy. Thus, the most likely explanation is that the process of discussing the symptoms with the nurse practitioner and feeling like they were being cared about, watched over, and given interventions improved how people felt, just like the workers in the Hawthorne plant worked harder knowing that they were being watched and that their managers were attempting to make their environment better.

If people feel better, are more productive, and work with higher quality after an intervention, is the Hawthorne effect a bad thing? Although in some cases the mere presence of the Hawthorne effect should not cause rejection of an intervention, there are several reasons to be cautious. First, Hawthorne effects tend to be temporary. Partly because high levels of observation are hard to maintain and partly because, as the saying goes, "culture trumps strategy," people tend to revert to their usual behavior over time. Second, repetitively trying new interventions can have diminishing returns. Eventually, instead of a Hawthorne effect, one will get a Dilbert effect, in which workers become skeptical and cynical about each new clever idea management has to increase quality or production. Third, resources are limited, so identifying the interventions and the parts of those interventions that really work allows efficient use of money, time, and energy.

Reference

1. Moeller AR, et al. Placard in hand: a simple, inexpensive intervention to improve on-treatment visit compliance in a safety net radiation oncology patient population. JCO Oncol Pract. 2020;16(11):e1272–81.
2. Mooney KH, et al. Automated home monitoring and management of patient-reported symptoms during chemotherapy: results of the symptom care at home RCT. Cancer Med. 2017;6(3):537–46.

Will Rogers Phenomenon

9

Will Rogers was born and raised in Oklahoma and became famous as a cowboy, actor, columnist, and humorist. He is known for his aphorisms, such as "I am not a member of any organized political party. I am a Democrat" or "Advertising is the art of convincing people to spend money they don't have for something they don't need," or "It isn't what we don't know that gives us trouble, it's what we know that ain't so." The Will Rogers phenomenon comes from one of his aphorisms about the place he grew up. During the Great Depression Dust Bowl, thousands of people left Oklahoma to move to California for jobs, a migration memorialized in John Steinbeck's *The Grapes of Wrath*. Will Rogers' comment was: "When the Okies left Oklahoma and moved to California, it raised the IQ of both states." What this means is that, in Rogers' opinion, the smartest people in California were not as smart as the least smart people in Oklahoma and that the smartest people stayed in Oklahoma. Thus, when the least smart people left Oklahoma, the average IQ in Oklahoma went up. Meanwhile, when they got to California, they were smarter than the people already there, so the average IQ in California went up. (Disclaimer: I am not endorsing his opinion about the relative intelligence of people in Oklahoma or California, merely summarizing it.) The Will Rogers phenomenon is when subgroups of a population are redefined so that the survival of all the subgroups increases while the survival of the entire population doesn't change.

The most common manifestation of the Will Rogers Phenomenon is stage migration. Stage refers to the extent of a cancer, i.e., how far it has spread. As technology changes over time, we get better at detecting small amounts of cancer spread throughout the body. Thus, people who previously had been called low stage get reclassified as high stage, changing the measured survival of both groups, despite the fact that no one lives any longer.

In addition, the definition of various stages changes over time. For example, in 2003, the standard staging system for cancers went from version 5 to version 6. For breast cancer, this change meant that women with four or more lymph nodes with cancer were automatically stage III whereas before they could be stage II or III. Thus, about half of women who would have been stage IIb in 2002 were stage

A. L. Cohen, *Problems and Pitfalls in Medical Literature*,
https://doi.org/10.1007/978-3-031-40295-1_9

III in 2003. Several papers showed that when women were reclassified using the 2003 system the survival rate of women with stage II and with stage III breast cancer both improved [1, 2]. For example, Tan et al. looked at women at the University of Malaya Medical Center with breast cancer [3]. Of these, 1230 were stage II under both the version 5 and version 6 systems, 511 were stage III under both systems, and 323 were stage II under version 5 but stage III under version 6. Using the old system, women with stage II breast cancer had a survival rate of 83% at 5 years and women with stage III breast cancer had a survival rate of 50% at 5 years. Using the new system to classify the same women, those with stage II breast cancer had a survival rate of 86% at 5 years and those with stage III breast cancer had a survival rate of 59% at 5 years. To use the Will Rogers analogy, the women with stage III breast cancer were in California, the women with stage II breast cancer were in Oklahoma, and by moving from stage II under the old system to stage III under the new system, survival was improved in both groups.

As a more subtle example, consider an article with the innocuous and seemingly self-evident title, "More extensive pelvic lymph node dissection improves survival in patients with node-positive prostate cancer" [4]. It seems like it should just make sense that if one does a better and more extensive surgery and removes more cancer to get a more accurate stage, people should live longer. However, there can be an apparent improvement in survival even if no one actually lives longer. Indeed, one should be wary because how can removing lymph nodes without cancer make people live longer. In this paper, the authors examined 315 people with pathologic N1 prostate cancer, meaning people who after surgery had prostate cancer found in their lymph nodes. They found that the number of lymph nodes removed was continuously related to survival. For example, people with 45 lymph nodes removed had a 97.9% chance of being alive 10 years later while people with 8 lymph nodes removed had a 74.7% chance of being alive 10 years later. Seems pretty convincing that one should remove 45 lymph nodes instead of 8.

The paper compares the survival of two groups of people: Group 1 is people who had 8 lymph nodes removed and Group 2 is people who had 45 lymph nodes removed (Fig. 9.1). However, there are really three groups of people here, not just two. Let's number the lymph nodes around the prostate 1–45 by the order in which they would be removed. (The numbering is a little contrived but gets the point

Fig. 9.1 Group breakdown for analysis of Will Roger effect

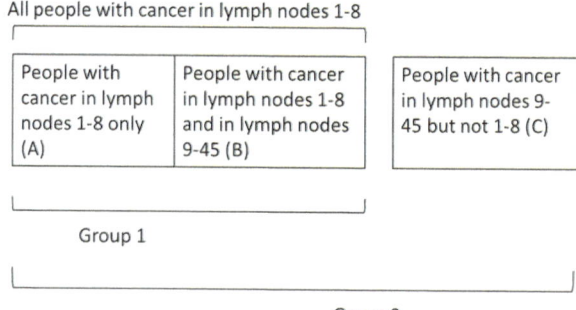

across.) Let's call Group A people with cancer in lymph nodes 1–8 but not lymph nodes 9–45; group B the people with cancer in lymph nodes 1–8 and in lymph nodes 9–45; and group C the people with lymph nodes 9–45 but not 1–8. Group 1 then consists of a mixture of Group B and Group A and Group 2 consists of a mixture of Group B and Group C. When we choose to remove 45 lymph nodes instead of 8, we are discovering the people in group C who would have been thought to not have cancer in their lymph nodes if only 8 nodes had been removed. The inclusion of group C improves the survival of group 2 compared to group 1 regardless of whether the surgery is actually beneficial. First, people with cancer in lymph nodes 1–8 and in 9–45 (group B) probably have more cancer overall than people who don't have cancer in nodes 1–8 for some reason. (Think about someone who has cancer in all 45 nodes compared to someone who just has cancer in node number 35.) Thus, the survival of group C is expected to be better than group B regardless of whether nodes are removed. Group C is the Okies moving to the California of Group B and raising the average survival. (Attentive readers may have also noticed there is some lead and length time bias going on as well but that's for another chapter.)

The real questions, then, are whether the survival of Group B is improved by surgery and whether the survival of Group C is improved by surgery, neither of which can be answered by retrospectively comparing the survival of Group A + B to Group A + B + C. Will Rogers strikes again.

References

1. Kim SI, Park BW, Lee KS. Comparison of stage-specific outcome of breast cancer based on 5th and 6th AJCC staging system. J Surg Oncol. 2006;93(3):221–7.
2. Woodward WA, et al. Changes in the 2003 American Joint Committee on Cancer staging for breast cancer dramatically affect stage-specific survival. J Clin Oncol. 2003;21(17):3244–8.
3. Tan GH, et al. The Will Rogers phenomenon in the staging of breast cancer - does it matter? Cancer Epidemiol. 2015;39(1):115–7.
4. Abdollah F, et al. More extensive pelvic lymph node dissection improves survival in patients with node-positive prostate cancer. Eur Urol. 2015;67(2):212–9.

Confounding occurs when one variable affects the relationship between the independent variable (the risk or intervention) and the dependent variable (outcome) without being the mechanism by which the independent variable influences the dependent variable. In other words, confounders are things that affect what you are trying to measure. Confounding can make relationships look stronger than they are in truth or weaker, depending on the circumstances. There are many forms of confounding, but we will focus on two. Confounding by severity, which is very similar to confounding by indication, is when people are assigned to intervention groups based on how sick they are/their individual risk of the outcome. Simpson's paradox occurs when the direction of an association is reversed when data are aggregated from different subgroups.

Confounding by Severity

10

Willie Sutton was a mid-twentieth century bank robber. Over the course of his life he stole over $2,000,000 from various banks. He eventually made it onto the FBIs 10-most wanted list. After he was captured, Willie Sutton was asked why he robbed banks. His answer, supposedly, was "Because that's where the money is." I like to think about Sutton's response in a bias known as confounding by severity.

Suppose you wanted to know where the most dangerous place in a hospital is. You could look at the death rate in various locations, including the cafeteria, registration, the ER, a medical floor, labor and delivery, and the ICU. If you did this exercise, you would find that the ICU is the most dangerous place with the highest death rates. Why? Because that's where the sicker people are. And, sicker people are more likely to die than less sick people. If you have pneumonia and it is recommended that you go to the ICU, should you refuse because the ICU has high death rates and the ICU kills people? No. The ICU has high death rates because people with severe diseases end up in the ICU and some of these die from their disease.

The above discussion is a reminder again of the mantra that correlation does not imply causation. When we look at studies that are not prospective intervention trials, mostly what we see are correlations. The goal of the reader, in these cases, should be to try to identify potential reasons for the correlation beside causation. These reasons are called confounders. Technically a confounder is a variable that has a causative relationship with both variables being studied whose presence or absence affects the correlation between those variables. In English confounders make it look like there is a relationship between two otherwise unrelated variables. There are many types of confounders. We will look at only a few of them, starting with confounding by severity.

The formal definition of confounding by severity is that it is a correlation between an intervention and an outcome that is determined by patient characteristics that correlate with both receiving (or not receiving) the intervention and the outcome. In other words, confounding by severity occurs because sicker people are more likely to get sicker than less sick people and people who are doing well are more likely to continue to do well. Another way to look at it is that many times we try to conclude

A. L. Cohen, *Problems and Pitfalls in Medical Literature*,
https://doi.org/10.1007/978-3-031-40295-1_10

that "all else being equal" some association or causation is true. Confounding by severity occurs when we try to compare groups where all else is *not* equal.

Confounding by severity can affect results in a couple of different ways. On the one hand, confounding by severity can make an intervention look less effective and/ or more dangerous than it is if that intervention is selectively done on people who are sick. For example, people who get complicated heart surgeries are more likely to die of heart disease than people who don't get complicated heart surgery, because you need to have pretty bad heart disease to need a complicated surgery. On the other hand, confounding by severity can make an intervention look more effective or more necessary than it is if it is selectively applied to people who are not too sick. In other words, if the only people who don't get surgery for appendicitis are those who are too sick from comorbidities and too close to death for surgery, then it will look like surgery is needed to prevent death from appendicitis whether that is true or not. Notice that in the first example (heart surgery) confounding by severity referred to the severity of the condition being intervened on (the heart disease) whereas in the second example (surgery for appendicitis) it referred to the severity of conditions unrelated to what was being intervened on.

Let's look at a couple of examples. As survival from breast cancer has improved, there has been great interest in trying to de-escalate therapy, i.e., maintain survival with less treatment. Thus, people have looked, particularly in older women, at whether there are groups of people who do not need various treatment modalities, including surgery, radiation, endocrine therapy, and chemotherapy. One such paper looked at women treated with lumpectomy for stage 1 breast cancer [1]. Standard of care in most of those women is radiation, though prospective trials have shown high survival rates in women over 70 with ER-positive tumors taking endocrine therapy who did not have radiation. The authors compared survival of women who received radiation versus those who did not. Out of nearly 7000 women, about 7% did not receive radiation. The survival of women who did not receive radiation (89% at 2 years) was significantly worse than those who did receive radiation (99% at 2 years). One possible interpretation is that rapid radiation is essential to convert incurable breast cancer into curable breast cancer. However, confounding by severity is a serious concern in these results.

Some people may have not received simply because they did not want radiation or because they or their physicians did not think they needed it. However, it is very likely that many people did not get radiation because they had serious health issues that made it unlikely they would live long enough to die of breast cancer. For those people we are confounding by the severity of their other diseases. Some evidence for this theory is that the rate of people with comorbidities was higher among people who did not receive radiation compared to people who received radiation (~20% vs ~14%), though knowing the percent with multiple comorbidities would strengthen this hypothesis. Ultimately, the proof would be seeing what people died from. If confounding by severity is the explanation, then most of the deaths would be expected to not be from breast cancer. Since it is hard to see how the receipt of breast radiation could prevent non-cancer deaths, if most of the deaths are due to other causes, that gives strong support to thinking that confounding by severity is the major contributor to the observed difference in survival. Unfortunately, data on whether someone dies is much easier to get than data on what they died from.

Interestingly, even people who died from breast cancer may still be examples of confounding by severity. Imagine someone who has surgery for what looks like a stage 1 breast cancer but who then has rapid recurrence and spread within a couple of months of what turned out to be a very aggressive breast cancer. Those people may have cancers so aggressive that they relapse before radiation can be done, and radiation would then not be done because it becomes futile. These cancers are aggressive enough that people are likely to die of them within the next 2 years. Although this may seem like immortal time bias, the difference is that here the death is still occurring after the radiation would have taken place, but the determination of whether to give the radiation or not is determined by factors that then go on to cause the death.

As another example, let's look at a situation where confounding by severity may make a treatment look less important than it probably is. Radiation is a standard therapy for glioblastoma, the deadly brain tumor. The standard paradigm when someone is diagnosed with a glioblastoma is that they have a surgery and then about 4 weeks later, when they have recovered from the surgery, they are treated with radiation. There have been a number of studies looking at what the optimal time to radiation treatment would be. One could hypothesize that earlier treatment would be better both for clinical and biologic reasons. On the other hand, if one could show that there was no advantage to earlier treatment, it allows greater flexibility and supports delaying treatment while screening for clinical trials.

Blumenthal et al. examine ~2800 people in a prospective database of people with newly diagnosed glioblastoma [2]. They divided the patients into four groups based on when they started radiation: <2 weeks, 2–3 weeks, 3–4 weeks, and >4 weeks. They then compared the survival among these four groups. Before we look at the results, let's think about what we might expect based on confounding by severity and other biases. We first have to think about why people might start radiation early or late. There are a couple of reasons that people would have been likely to start radiation earlier. The first is that people who have unresectable tumors that are diagnosed by biopsy do not have large incisions that need to heal so can start earlier, but these are also tumors with poorer prognosis due to not being resectable. The second is that doctors are more likely to expedite radiation in people who are sicker and whom the doctors believe are at higher risk for earlier tumor progression. Therefore, we have a good setup for confounding by severity, whereby people who have worse tumors and who are sicker get radiation earlier and are also more likely to die earlier based on their disease, which would be expected to make earlier radiation appear more deadly than later radiation.

In fact, that's exactly what they saw. The median survival for people who received radiation in less than 2 weeks was 9.2 months compared to 12.5 months for people who received radiation more than 4 weeks after surgery. The survival for people who received radiation 2–3 weeks or 3–4 weeks after surgery was in between. Due to the large number of patients, these differences were statistically significant. These differences are likely due to confounding by severity.

There is one other bias that may be affecting these results, which falls more into the category of selection bias, with some component of immortal time bias. All of the patients in this study received radiation. Thus, if someone had surgery and had symptomatic tumor progression 5 weeks later that led to rapid decompensation and death, they were not included, but if that same person started radiation 3 weeks after surgery and avoided the progression, then they were included. This difference also leads to a bias toward longer survival for people who start radiation later.

How does one avoid confounding by severity? The best way is prospective randomization, which both facilitates balancing of potentially confounding variable including disease severity and avoids having physicians subconsciously or consciously assigning patients to treatments based on severity. In a retrospective trial it is difficult to completely exclude confounding by severity. Several methods can be used to help. All are based on the idea of trying to ensure that groups are as balanced as possible based on potentially confounding variables, particularly those related to severity. A common way of doing this is propensity matching. Propensity matching decreases the sample size by picking a subset of patients that are well matched by the variables of interest. The success of propensity scoring is highly affected by how well the variables picked for matching encompass the range of severity of the disease.

References

1. Bazan JG, et al. De-escalation of radiation therapy in patients with stage I, node-negative, HER2-positive breast cancer. NPJ Breast Cancer. 2021;7(1):33.
2. Blumenthal DT, et al. Short delay in initiation of radiotherapy may not affect outcome of patients with glioblastoma: a secondary analysis from the radiation therapy oncology group database. J Clin Oncol. 2009;27(5):733–9.

Simpson's Paradox

11

Suppose you wanted to know if we are winning the war on cancer. Put aside the important question of why we use military analogies for these sorts of things or what it even means to declare war on a disease, particularly a non-infectious one. Let's just ask whether the risk of dying from cancer is going down over time. If we compare how many people died from cancer in the US in 2020 compared to 1990 we would find that more people died of cancer in 2020. It's pretty easy to see that such a comparison is unfair, however, because there are more people in the US in 2020 than in 1990, about 50 million more. So, the first adjustment one must make is to look at the rate of cancer death per person, or more traditionally per 100,000 people. By this measure, the numbers still don't look good. The death rate from cancer has increased by about 20%, from 212/100,000 people in 1990 to 236/100,000 people in 2020. With all of our screening, knowledge of healthy behavior, and cool new treatments, what gives?

What gives is there is one more important variable to look at: age. Cancer is a disease of aging and between 1990 and 2020 the average age of the US population increased. If we crudely divide the population at 55, we see that in people under 55, the death rate from cancer decreased by 20%, going from 52/100,000 people to 43/100,000 and in people over 55 the death rate from cancer decreased by 20% going from 892/100,000 to 733/100,000. In other words, a young person is 20% less likely to die of cancer in 2020 compared to 1990 and an older person is 20% less likely to die of cancer in 2020 than in 1990, but a random person in the population is 20% more likely to die of cancer. How can that be? (One may wonder if the problem is because of my arbitrary choice of 55 to divide young and old people. There are real and important issues with dichotomizing a continuous variable so it should not be done lightly or capriciously. Although I did it here for the sake of narrative simplicity, the trends hold regardless of the cutoff or if one does the proper continuous age adjustment.)

The explanation is that, in addition to the population growing, the population is getting older over time. The average age in the US is rising over time. The total rate of cancer death is a weighted combination of the rate of cancer death in the young

© The Author(s), under exclusive license to Springer Nature Switzerland AG 2023   47
A. L. Cohen, *Problems and Pitfalls in Medical Literature*,
https://doi.org/10.1007/978-3-031-40295-1_11

and the rate of cancer death in the older population, weighted by how many people are in each group. Thus, even though the rates in both groups are going down over time, because there are more people in the older group, the overall population average is getting closer to that higher figure.

The situation where trends in subgroups are reversed when looking at the entire population is called Simpson's paradox. Simpson's paradox occurs when the relationship between two variables is reversed or negated when going from looking at an entire population to looking at subgroups. So, a particular diet could be good for women, good for men, but look bad in the overall population. Or, an athlete could outperform another athlete each year but look worse when multiple years are combined. Simpson's paradox comes up when aggregating data. Simpson's paradox is related to confounding because the variable that defines the subgroup is a confounder.

The difficulty with Simpson's paradox is knowing when it is a factor. Sometimes it is obvious that data is being aggregated, say if several different centers or different countries are involved in a study. There are also commonly defined subgroups, such as those by age or gender, that should always be checked. Other times, it may not be obvious without specialized knowledge what subgroups to consider.

For example, in acute myeloid leukemia (AML), prognosis is often driven by mutations in the tumor cells. In a study illustrating Simpson's paradox, researchers looked at mutations in a gene called DNMT3A. Overall, looking at everyone with AML, the presence of mutations in DNMT3A is not prognostic. However, researchers also looked at another important gene, NPM1. When NPM1 is mutated, then the presence of DNMT3A mutations decreases survival by about 20%. When NPM1 is not mutated, the presence of DNMT3A decreases survival by about 40% [1].

How do you know, then, if you have looked at enough variables and subgroups to be confident that Simpson's paradox is not happening? In some ways, there is no test and one can never be sure, so it's easy to get paranoid that Simpson's paradox could always be lurking. The best you can do is think deeply about what variables could explain the outcome and check results in the subgroups that are common and those that make biologic sense in the question being asked. What you want to look for are tables or graphs, a Forrest plot being one example, where results are given in several subgroups defined by geography, gender, ethnicity, or biology to see if there is consistency in the results in all of them. If no issues are seen in any of those, then it becomes less likely there is some hidden lurking variable out there that will reverse results. However, Simpson's paradox reminds us to be humble about the effects of the so-called unknown unknowns.

Reference

1. Gale RE, et al. Simpson's paradox and the impact of different DNMT3A mutations on outcome in younger adults with acute myeloid leukemia. J Clin Oncol. 2015;33(18):2072–83.

Part IV

Misuse of Tests

When statistical tests are not used the way they were developed and intended, false or misleading results can occur. Using hypothesis testing procedures without a clear hypothesis can lead to false beliefs. In particular, when many tests are done on the same data, there will be some "statistically significant" associations just by chance. Proper correction must be made for such multiple comparisons, and one must remember that they are hypothesis generating only. Similarly, results for predefined primary endpoints should be considered more convincing than results for secondary endpoints or endpoints added after the study is completed. Predictive models should be validated in external datasets before they are accepted. In survival analysis, measures that average over the whole curve, such as the hazard ratio, should only be used when curves are parallel, i.e., the proportional hazard assumption is satisfied. We look at examples of studies that have done too many tests, also called data mining or p-hacking, have reported endpoints that were not prespecified, have not validated models on external datasets, and computed hazard ratios that are meaningless.

Multiple Comparisons

12

We all know the adage "If at first you don't succeed, try, try again." Although there are many places that this wisdom applies, statistical testing is not one of them. The problem with "try, try again" is that the more one tries, the more likely one is to find random things that don't mean anything. When one asks a question and has a guess for the answer, that is a hypothesis. Data can then be used to support or refute that hypothesis. When one looks at data without a pre-existing question or guess, then that is "hypothesis generation," which can be important but should never be taken as definitive.

When I was in elementary school, lists would go around purporting to prove that John F Kennedy was the reincarnation of Abraham Lincoln based on certain similarities. Kennedy and Lincoln both have seven letters. Both were elected to Congress in a year ending in 46 and to the presidency in a year ending in 60. Both were assassinated in office. Lincoln was assassinated in a theater and the assassin fled to a warehouse. Kennedy was assassinated in a warehouse and the assassin fled to a theater. Etc.

The problem with this line of thinking is that you can take any two people and find a list of "eerie" similarities if you are willing to consider enough variables. Suppose I wanted to prove Bill Clinton and Grover Cleveland were somehow karmically linked. Both were elected in years ending in 92. Both names start with Cl. Both were governors before becoming president. Both were criticized for avoiding the draft. Both had sex scandals while in office. Cleveland married a woman 27 years younger than him. Clinton had an affair with a woman 27 years younger than him. I could go on but you can get the point. These similarities don't mean anything more than the observation that presidents elected in years ending in zero are more likely to be shot than other presidents (5 out of 11 vs 1 out of 31, $p = 0.00058$). When one computes enough p-values then one out of 20 is going to be less than 0.05 (statistically significant) just by chance. This problem is called multiple comparisons.

Multiple comparisons can show up in a few different ways. The most obvious is when a paper includes a large number of tests and then focuses on the ones with low p-values. Retrospective analyses of large datasets often have this problem. Consider,

© The Author(s), under exclusive license to Springer Nature Switzerland AG 2023
A. L. Cohen, *Problems and Pitfalls in Medical Literature*,
https://doi.org/10.1007/978-3-031-40295-1_12

for example, a paper with a title such as "Increased Acid-Producing Diet and Past Smoking Intensity Are Associated with Worse Prognoses among Breast Cancer Survivors: A Prospective Cohort Study," published in the *Journal of Clinical Medicine* in June of 2020. By the title alone, there are two possibilities for how an association between dietary acid, smoking, and breast cancer could have been identified. One is that there were pre-existing data in other cohorts and biologic mechanism studies suggested an association that this study was attempting to confirm independently. The second, more likely scenario, is that the authors set out to look at dietary acid in this cohort, found that it did not predict survival, and then looked at a bunch of variables and subgroups until they found one (namely smokers) where such an association is seen. In the second case, the association is interesting and may be worth future study but has a high chance of being random and should not be taken too seriously unless it is confirmed in other settings.

Multiple comparison issues can creep into prospective clinical trials as well. In this setting, one should watch for authors focusing on a secondary endpoint when the primary endpoint was not significant. As an example, consider "Memantine for the prevention of cognitive dysfunction in patients receiving whole-brain radiotherapy: a randomized, double-blind, placebo-controlled trial" [1]. Whole brain radiation is a treatment used when someone has enough spots of cancer in their brain that doing more focused treatments is not feasible. Whole brain radiation is very effective at controlling cancer. The problem with whole brain radiation is that the normal brain doesn't particularly like being radiated, so people who have whole brain radiation can develop cognitive problems, including memory problems, slow thinking, trouble concentrating, etc. At its worst, a full-blown dementia can develop. Therefore, scientists have studied ways to try to prevent thinking problems in people who receive whole brain radiation. Memantine is a drug used in Alzheimer's disease that seems to slow down cognitive decline in people with that disease, so it was natural to test in people with whole brain radiation.

In the trial, 508 people were enrolled and all received standard whole brain radiation. Participants were randomly assigned to take memantine during and after the radiation or to take a placebo. A battery of tests was given to people at the beginning of the trial and then 4 more times over the next year. The primary endpoint of the study was memory (measured by a test called HVLT-R DR) at 24 weeks after the radiation. This means that the study was designed to test a hypothesis about this particular test. The size of the study was determined based on a goal change in this test. So, before the trial started, the planners of the trial thought the most important outcome and the one most representative of the effects of this drug was HVLT-R DR results 24 weeks after radiation. In total, though, there were 8 tests (6 different tests, one of which has two subtests, and a composite of all the test) that have raw and standardized scores measured at 4 different time points and analyzed both at the specified time points and as time to significant decrease. Thus, in all there were 90 different variables being looked at.

The primary outcome of the study was not statistically significant. As with all results that are not statistically significant this result could mean that the drug does not work or that the study did not have enough power to detect the amount that it worked. Either way, there is not definitive evidence that memantine has a clinically meaningful effect on delaying memory loss in people who have whole brain radiation. How then did the authors conclude that memantine resulted in "better cognitive function over time" leading to the use of memantine in guidelines and future trials?

Of the 90 possible tests done, statistical significance was reached in five of them identified in the paper. Many of the other tests "trended" toward improvement in the memantine arm, meaning the people who took memantine were a little better, but the differences were not statistically significant. If one is being generous, one can conclude that there may be a small benefit to memantine that this study was not powered enough to show and that this difference may show up in different tests in different people. The less generous interpretation is that there is no difference and the few low p-values are pretty much due to random chance. I'd come down in between, thinking there is probably a small difference with memantine but that it is small enough that I wouldn't hang my hat on it or think it is clinically important.

There's a lot of controversy about when multiple comparisons are a problem and how to deal with it. For example, some large datasets have been studied over and over by many groups over the years. If each research group only looks at five variables but there are 100 different research groups, should we think of that as really being 500 variables? The true answer is probably that it depends, but it is important to know there is not one simple answer.

To compensate for multiple comparisons, some argue it is best to just acknowledge the potential issue, be very explicit about whether a study is hypothesis-generating or trying to definitively evaluate a hypothesis, and move on. Others suggest that to avoid false-positive statistical significance one should adjust the p-value one considers statistically significant. There are different rules for how to do this adjustment. The simplest is called the Bonferroni correction. For the Bonferroni correction, one divides the goal p-value (usually 0.05) by the number of variable. So, if one is doing 100 tests, then significance is declared if the p-value is less than 0.05 divided by 100, which is 0.0005. The tradeoff is that the power goes down when one does such a correction. The Bonferroni correction is commonly used and cited, but it is important to remember that, like any other tool, it is neither intrinsically right nor wrong and deliberation is needed about what is best in any given situation.

Reference

1. Brown PD, et al. Memantine for the prevention of cognitive dysfunction in patients receiving whole-brain radiotherapy: a randomized, double-blind, placebo-controlled trial. Neuro-Oncology. 2013;15(10):1429–37.

Validation

13

Science in general and medical science in particular is a voyage of discovery. Sometimes, one has a hypothesis based on prior research that leads to an experiment that gets written up and published. Sometimes, however, we don't yet know what we are looking for. We want to predict some good or bad thing to help people prepare to make decisions. Those predictions are often complicated. For example, we may want to predict how long someone is likely to live to decide whether doing surgery for a tumor is worthwhile. Many factors could go into that prediction, such as how old someone is, what health conditions they have, how good their diet is, whether they smoke, etc. In such a situation, we need a mathematical model to incorporate and weigh all of these factors to make the prediction.

There are many ways to make a mathematical model for prediction. These include relatively straightforward techniques such as logistic regression to complicated and fancy artificial intelligence techniques involving machine learning or neural networks. It can seem like every year there is some cool new technology that is supposed to take giant amounts of data and analyze it to give us the answers we want. Understanding these technologies is hard. Fortunately, understanding whether they are useful is less hard.

All models begin in a process called development. Development involves building a model by designating a set of variables to look at and having a dataset where those variables are known about the people in that dataset and the outcome of interest is also known about those people. The model then does its magic, which for this discussion we don't care about, to pick some of those variables and assign them weights based on how important they are to determine a formula that takes in the values of those variables and spits out a prediction. Depending on the technology, one could end up with two variables or with thousands of variables. It doesn't matter as long as it spits out a prediction.

As an example, we'll consider a paper on predicting early-onset colon cancer [1]. Note that I'm not trying to single out this paper, and there are a million other similar papers I could have picked that all illustrate the same points. In this paper, the authors wanted to predict based on variables in an electronic health record whether someone's colonoscopy would show cancer or not. They started with a dataset of 3116 people. They looked at about 50 variables. They used various methods to then build their final model. They then applied the model to the dataset they had and showed that it was 96% accurate, which sounds pretty good.

Once the model is built, we need to test the model. There are a number of tests that are used for assessing how good a model fits data, including the C-index or the area under the receiver operator curve (AUC). The important thing is not the test used, however. The important thing is the dataset on which the model is tested.

The easiest thing is to see how good the prediction is in the dataset used to develop the model. This step is called internal validation. As you can imagine, if a model doesn't look good on internal validation, it is a really bad model and should get thrown out. On the other hand, if a model looks good on internal validation, don't get too impressed. Remember that for internal validation, the model was built on that dataset, so the model was specifically constructed to fit the data in that dataset. It is thus somewhat circular to then declare success because the model fits the data in that dataset. Because of issues similar to what was discussed in the multiple comparison chapter, with enough variables, one can always find a model that fits a given dataset, particularly if the number of variables one is looking at is comparable to or more than the number of people in the dataset. This situation leads to a problem called overfitting.

In our paper above, notice that the cancer prediction model was developed and tested on the same dataset. Given that the model was derived to fit this dataset, it should not come as a surprise that it is very accurate in this dataset. That accuracy does not, in and of itself, however, give great confidence that the model will work in any other dataset. Other datasets may give different results for various reasons. Sometimes, a model performs differently in different datasets because of actual differences between populations. A model built in men might not work in women. A model built in Europe might not work in the US where the diet is different. These problems are why facial recognition systems that were primarily built using databases of young white Americans perform poorly in other groups, for example. Sometimes, a model performs differently because data is structured differently. For example, the colon cancer prediction model might have trouble if smoking is recorded as pack-years in some electronic health systems and as yes/no in other health systems. Lastly, a model might perform differently just because of random chance.

When one only has a single dataset to work with, there are a couple of ways to try to account for overfitting. The first is called cross validation. In cross validation, one takes out some of the data from the dataset and rederives the model to check to make sure it doesn't change much, i.e., that it is not too dependent on small changes in the dataset. Cross validation is nice but is the least one can do and should not give too much confidence. The second involves splitting the dataset. Typically, the dataset is split into a development group of about 2/3 to 3/4 of the group and a validation group with the rest of the subjects. The model is then built in the development group and tested for accuracy in the validation group. Splitting helps reduce the chance of random effects, but it does not help with the issue of differing demographics or different data structures mentioned above.

The gold standard for testing a model is called external validation. External validation is when a model is tested in a completely different dataset than the one on which it was built. The more different the dataset and the more different datasets that are used for external validation the better. When assessing a prediction model, one should always look for external validation. If it is not present, the model should be considered interesting but not ready for primetime, like the colon cancer prediction model above. Once a model has been externally validated in a diverse array of settings, it is likely good to use.

Reference

1. Hussan H, et al. Utility of machine learning in developing a predictive model for early-age-onset colorectal neoplasia using electronic health records. PLoS One. 2022;17(3):e0265209.

Proportional Hazard Violation

14

Time-dependent endpoints are those measures that look at how long it takes within a group for some event to happen. If we want to look at how long people live with a certain disease, then we measure the time to the event of death and call it overall survival. If we want to look at how long after a surgery it will take for a tumor to regrow, then we measure the time to the event of recurrence of the tumor and call it recurrence-free survival. If we want to know how long someone's quality of life is going to be good, then we measure the time to the event defined by the threshold on some quality of life measure, and we may call that measurement time until clinical decline.

Time-dependent endpoints are often expressed as medians or percentages at a specific time, e.g., one-year survival or progression-free survival at 6 months, or fancy measures like the restricted mean survival time, which is a way to take an average despite having some people in a study who have not had an event. Visually, we depict time-dependent measures as survival curves. In a typical survival curve, the horizontal (x-axis) is time, and the vertical (y-axis) is the probability of not having reached the event. At the top of the y-axis is 1, or 100%, meaning 100% of people have not reached the event. (Using death as the event of interest, for example, this means we start the study with nobody having died yet, which is generally a good idea.) The bottom of the y-axis is 0, which means everyone has reached the event. Over the course of the study, the survival curve starts at the upper left point, coordinates (0,1) meaning time 0 and 100% survival, and moves down and to the right as time passes and people experience whatever event is being studied.

In most research studies involving survival data, we want to know if two groups have different survival, i.e., we need to compare two different survival curves. One way to do this is to simply ask if two curves are different, which we do by comparing the survival across the whole curves. The test that does this comparison is called the log-rank test. The log-rank test gives a yes/no answer to the question, "are these two survival curves significantly different?" It doesn't tell how they are different or how much they are different. For those we need a measure that looks at whether one curve decreases faster than the other.

© The Author(s), under exclusive license to Springer Nature Switzerland AG 2023

A. L. Cohen, *Problems and Pitfalls in Medical Literature*,

https://doi.org/10.1007/978-3-031-40295-1_14

The speed at which the survival curve decreases over time is called the hazard rate. This concept of the rate of change of a curve may be giving you flashbacks to calculus class. If you are interested in the technical details you would need calculus, but thankfully we don't need to go there. Take a deep breath. Have no fear. I promised no formulas and am keeping that promise. To be precise, a curve can have different hazard rates at each point in time. However, dealing with all of the hazard rates over time gets really complicated, so usually we just look at the average hazard rate over the course of the curve.

To compare the speed at which two curves decrease over time, we want to compare their hazard rates. To compare the average hazard rates for two curves, we divide one hazard rate by another to get a hazard ratio. Thus, if the hazard ratio is 1.5, it means one curve is decreasing 50% faster than the other. The important thing about the hazard ratio is that it is one number that summarizes the comparison of how fast the curves decrease across the whole curves. So, the hazard ratio only makes sense if the rate at which the curves decrease over time has the same pattern for each curve. The most simple (and common) way they can have the same pattern is if both curves have a constant hazard rate. So, if one group has a rate of 2 events per month and the other group has a rate of 3 events per month and these don't change much month to month, then it is pretty easy to say that the hazard ratio should be 1.5, which is three divided by two. Another way they can have the same pattern is if the hazard rate changes in the same way over time. So, if one group has a rate of 4 events per month for 6 months and then 2 events per month and the other group has a rate of 6 events per month and then 3 events per month, then the hazard ratio is still 1.5. The assumption that the pattern of hazard rate is changing the same way over time between two curves is called the proportional hazard assumption. Another way to think about the proportional hazard assumption is that two curves have proportional hazards if they are approximately parallel over most of their course.

We run into trouble when trying to use an average measure like the hazard ratio to compare curves that are not parallel, i.e., where the proportional hazard ratio is not valid. When proportional hazard assumption is violated, then the hazard ratio is not meaningful. As a number it can still be calculated, meaning you can plug numbers into the formula and get a number out without exploding whatever calculator or computer you is using. You can put that number on a graph and publish it. However, just because you can calculate it, that doesn't mean you should. It doesn't mean anything. Consider two basketball teams. One wins every game in the first half of the season and loses every game in the second half of the season. The other loses every game in the first half of the season and wins every game in the second half of the season. Both teams won half their games. However, it would not be meaningful to say they had equivalent seasons.

In medicine, the proportional hazard assumption tends to be violated when there are unidentified confounders or subgroups within the population. Rather than ignore this possibility and focus on a meaningless hazard ratio number, the better approach is to try to identify the unidentified confounder. Using the basketball analogy above, rather than saying that both teams have a record of 0.500, we should be asking what happened with each team at the halfway point.

For an example, consider the IPASS trial, which was published in the *New England Journal of Medicine* in 2009 [1]. In the early 2000s, the standard treatment for lung cancer was chemotherapy. It was found that the protein EGFR was important in many lung adenocarcinomas, a common type of lung cancer in people in Asia and people who were not heavy smokers. Therefore, people studied drugs that blocked EGFR as treatments for lung cancer. IPASS compared gefitinib, which is an EGFR inhibitor, with carboplatin-paclitaxel, which is a chemotherapy combination, in the treatment of lung adenocarcinoma. The study concluded that "gefitinib is superior to carboplatin-paclitaxel" based on a hazard ratio for progression-free survival of 0.74, $p < 0.001$.

The figure shows the survival curves for the two groups (Fig. 14.1). The first observation that should be readily apparent is that the two curves are not parallel. The gefitinib curve drops at a fairly steady pace the whole time while the chemotherapy curve is slower at first then drops quickly at about 6 months and then slows down again. In other words, there appear to be two groups of people. In one group, their lung cancer progresses quickly, and they do better with chemotherapy. In the second group, their cancers progress more slowly, and they do better with gefitinib. Thus, although the curves are clearly different, it is not meaningful to say that gefitinib is 26% better than chemotherapy. Rather, what's meaningful is to conclude that for some people, chemotherapy is better and for some people gefitinib is better. The average benefit will then depend on the number of each type of person in the sample, which requires figuring out who those people are. The better way to analyze the data would have been to do a log-rank test to show that the curves were significantly different and then say that a hazard ratio was not computed due to lack of proportional hazards.

It turns out that after the study started but before it was published, scientists figured out that in some lung cancers, particularly in Asians and non-smokers, that EGFR protein is mutated. When the authors looked at the IPASS population, EGFR mutation defined the two populations (Fig. 14.2). When EGFR mutation is present,

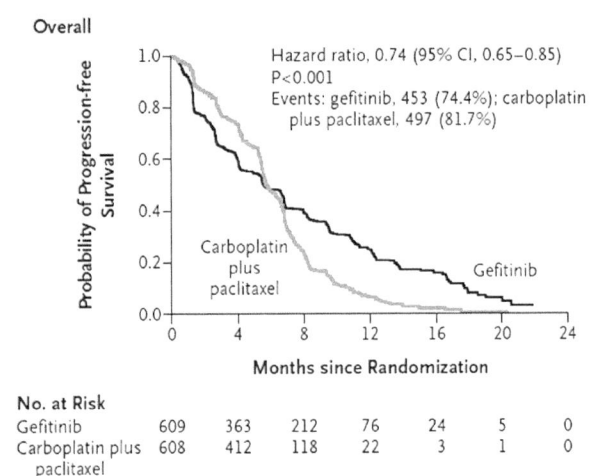

Fig. 14.1 Example of a survival curve showing lack of proportional hazards

Fig. 14.2 Subgroup
analysis showing the
reason for loss of
proportional hazards

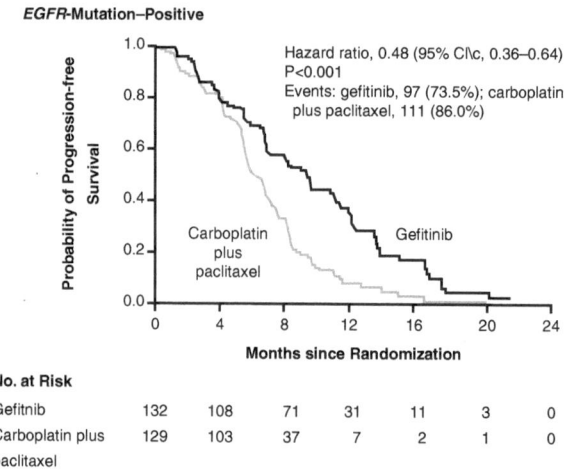

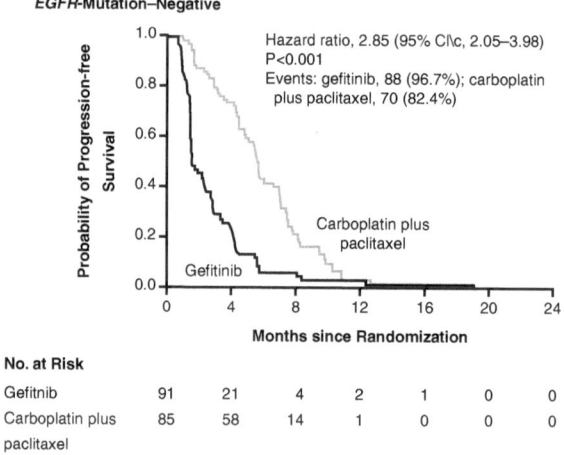

the proportional hazard assumption is satisfied, and gefitinib is superior to chemotherapy with a hazard ratio of 0.48. When EGFR is not present, the proportional
hazard assumption is satisfied, and gefitinib is inferior to chemotherapy with a hazard ratio of 2.85.

There are two morals to the IPASS study. The first is that looking at the images
of the survival curves often tells you more than reading the abstract of a study. The
second is to be aware of the assumptions underlying tests or summary statistics,
particularly when an entire distribution is being summarized in one number.

Reference

1. Mok TS, et al. Gefitinib or carboplatin-paclitaxel in pulmonary adenocarcinoma. N Engl J
   Med. 2009;361(10):947–57.

Changing Endpoints

15

There is a fable about a storyteller who always had the right story for any occasion. One day a child asks her how she always knew a story that was such a good fit for the situation. The storyteller replied, of course, with a story. Once there was an archer who was known far and wide for always hitting the center of a bullseye. People from all over the land would talk about how they had seen bullseyes with his arrows sticking out of the middle. When he was on his deathbed, someone asked him what his secret to archery was. He said, "First, I fire the arrow. Then, I paint the target." Knowing whether the target was painted before or after the arrow was fired is essential for interpreting scientific studies.

Every scientific study starts with a question and a hypothesis about what the answer to that question is. The investigator then decides how they will answer the question. The question becomes the primary objective of the study, and the measure that will be used to answer it is the primary endpoint. The question, hypothesis, primary objective, and primary endpoint are laid out ahead of time, which is necessary to the assumptions underlying the statistical analysis if we want to test the hypothesis and draw a conclusion.

Sometimes, one starts out a study not having an idea what one will find. In that case, the study is called hypothesis generating because one is using the study to generate a hypothesis. Hypothesis generating studies are important, but they should never be considered definitive, for all the reasons discussed in the chapter on multiple comparisons.

Studies always look at more than one question in the end. Questions that the study intends to look at that are not the primary objective are called secondary objectives. Secondary objectives may be questions that are considered less important than the primary objective or may be questions that the current study is too small to really answer but it can give some information on. Thus, secondary objectives are usually either hypothesis generating or questions the study is underpowered to answer with any precision. Secondary objectives are stated before the study started, so they carry more weight than questions that are raised after looking at the data, which are called post-hoc analyses and are purely hypothesis generating.

© The Author(s), under exclusive license to Springer Nature Switzerland AG 2023
A. L. Cohen, *Problems and Pitfalls in Medical Literature*,
https://doi.org/10.1007/978-3-031-40295-1_15

Nonetheless, secondary objectives are rarely answered definitively in a study and should be validated in separate studies. Unfortunately, sometimes results about secondary objectives can be so seductive that they become the focus of attention beyond the primary objectives.

In 2010, the *New England Journal of Medicine* published a randomized trial on early palliative care in people with metastatic lung cancer [1]. The patients were randomized soon after diagnosis to either usual care or to usual care plus meetings with a palliative care physician focused on symptom management. The primary objective was to measure quality of life using a scale called the Trial Outcome Index (TOI). The TOI is a scale from 0 to 84, where higher numbers mean better quality of life. The patients who were assigned to meet with a palliative care provider did end up with better quality of life, with an average score of 59 out of 84 compared to 53 out of 84, which is a real difference that was statistically significant and would be considered moderately sized statistically and a small clinical improvement.

What got the paper into the top medical journal in the country though was that the group that was assigned to meet with a palliative care provider also lived longer, with half of people still alive at 11.6 months compared to 8.9 months in the usual care group. Such a result is intriguing and ended up changing practice and guidelines across the country. To understand its validity, however, we need to look deeper at the trial design.

Like many good journals, the *NEJM* has taken to publishing the protocol when they publish an article, in part to help readers compare what is presented to what the authors said they were going to do. In this case, the protocol includes the objectives of the study. Survival was not the primary objective of the study. It was not even a secondary objective of the study. It was either a completely post-hoc analysis or thought to be so unlikely to show a difference that it was not included in the original study design.

Because of the risk of multiple comparisons and random false positives, particularly in small studies, an unplanned and unexpected result like this should be considered hypothesis generating rather than hypothesis confirming. It requires validation, which will never occur, unfortunately. There is no doubt that early attention to symptoms and quality of life in people with incurable cancer is a good thing, but we will never know if it really makes people live longer. Indeed, when people have looked in other cancer types, no such improvement has been seen.

Being on the lookout for whether an article is focused on the primary objective or other preplanned analysis or a post-hoc analysis is important for assessing studies. Sometimes, the text of an article will tell you, but often, particularly when the primary objective is a negative result but something else looks really cool, the focus may be completely shifted to a new objective. That's when comparing against a published protocol, looking at prior articles about the study, or reviewing clinical trial registries such as clinicaltrials.gov is helpful to understand whether a result is definitive or merely hypothesis generating.

Reference

1. Temel JS, et al. Early palliative care for patients with metastatic non-small-cell lung cancer. N Engl J Med. 2010;363(8):733–42.

Part V

Power

Power refers to the chance of detecting a particular outcome if that outcome is true. Power is related to the sample size of a study and the size of the outcome being studied. Underpowered studies are too small and risk false-negative results, also called type II errors, in which a true effect is missed. Overpowered studies are too large and risk detecting small but meaningless effects. The size of the effect being aimed for in a study, which then determines the sample size for a given power, should be based on clinical judgment not simply availability of resources. We look at examples of overpowered and underpowered studies.

Underpowering

16

As we all know, it's very hard to prove a negative. In statistics, the formal way of saying that is that we never can accept the null hypothesis, which typically is that two groups are the same. We can only say that we have not proven they are different and that it is unlikely they are very different. Power is one of the concepts related to what we mean by "unlikely" and "very different."

The size of a study is inextricably linked to how big an effect we are trying to detect, the false-positive rate we are willing to accept, and the false-negative rate we are willing to accept. Critics of evidence-based medicine like to raise a strawman argument by asking in a sarcastic tone why practitioners of evidence-based medicine don't insist on and volunteer for placebo-controlled, randomized control trials of parachutes when jumping out of a plane. In truth, this situation is just an extreme example of the effects of effect size, false-positive rate, and false-negative rate on sample size. When jumping out of an airplane, we are looking for a big effect (100% survival versus essentially 0% survival) while accepting a high false-positive rate (we don't mind using extra unnecessary precautions) and high false-negative rate (as long as something works we don't mind not using other precautions that might also work) which leads to a very low sample size needed; in this case 1 person who uses a parachute and survives is enough.

Most of the time, however, we are not dealing with such an extreme situation. Even incurable cancers have outliers who unexplainably live a long time, and most treatments are not 100% effective. Thus, most questions require randomized studies with sample sizes much larger than one. When designing a study, we don't have much control over the effect size we want to see, which is determined by the needs of the community with that disease (a topic for the next chapter). We also don't have much control over the false-positive rate, which for better or worse (and there has been much written about why it is for the worse) has been traditionally set at 5% or 0.05. Thus, the biggest way to affect the sample size is by changing the false-negative rate.

The inverse of the false-negative rate is power. So power is 100% minus the false-negative rate. If the false-negative rate is 10%, then the power is 90%. If the

© The Author(s), under exclusive license to Springer Nature Switzerland AG 2023
A. L. Cohen, *Problems and Pitfalls in Medical Literature*,
https://doi.org/10.1007/978-3-031-40295-1_16

false-negative rate is 25%, then the power is 75%. Officially, power is the probability of detecting a difference (having a positive study) if there really is a difference. Power, then, is related to sample size. With a big sample size, the false-negative rate is small and power is high. With a small sample size, the false-negative rate is large and power is low. Studies can run into trouble by having too little power (underpowered studies) or having too much power (overpowered studies). In the next chapter we'll talk about overpowered studies. In this chapter, we will discuss underpowered studies.

As the previous paragraph indicates, power mostly comes into play when a study is negative, i.e., when it does not show a significant difference between groups. When a study is negative, the correct interpretation is not that the two groups are equal. The correct interpretation is that either the two groups are equal or the study was too small (underpowered) to distinguish the true difference between the groups.

As an example, consider the example of postoperative chemotherapy for non-small cell lung cancer (NSCLC). NSCLC is the most common cancer in the United States and the most common cause of cancer death. More women die of NSCLC than of breast cancer. More men die of NSCLC than of prostate cancer. In short, NSCLC is bad and common. When NSCLC is caught early (stage I-II), all visible tumor can be removed by surgery. Although some people can be cured this way, most people have recurrence within a few years and ultimately die from the NSCLC. Therefore, people have been studying for decades about what to do after surgery to reduce the chance that the NSCLC comes back and thus to cure more people.

In the late 1990s and early 2000s, several groups did clinical trials comparing chemotherapy to no chemotherapy after surgery for early stage NSCLC. One such trial was CALGB 9633, so named because it started in 1996 [1]. In this study, 344 people with resected stage 1B NSCLC were randomized after surgery to chemotherapy (carboplatin and paclitaxel) or no chemotherapy. After 5 years, 60% of people who got chemotherapy were alive and 58% of people who did not get chemotherapy were alive, and the difference in overall survival was not significant with a p-value of 0.125. Should we conclude that chemotherapy does not work?

Looking at the statistical analysis section of the paper, we see that the study was originally designed to recruit 500 people to have an 80% power to detect an increase in 5-year survival from 50% to 63% with a 2-sided p-value of 0.05. However, because they were only able to recruit 344 people and the survival in the control group was higher than expected, the true power of the study was lower than the planned 80%. (Technical point that can be ignored if it bores you: The study team attempted to compensate for this problem with longer follow-up and changing from a 2-tailed test to 1-tailed test, which allows the ostensible power to remain at 80% but when looking at 5-year survival rather than hazard ratio the length of follow-up is less important and the change to 1-tailed test in the middle of the study was really just an admission that the power was decreased.) Thus, with a study this size, there was at least a 20% and probably more like 30% or higher chance of a negative study even if there is a 13% absolute benefit from chemotherapy. Thus, in an underpowered study like this, the chance of a false negative is not low.

Was this a false-negative study? The answer is probably. Ultimately, there were 6 randomized trials done of chemotherapy for NSCLC combined into a meta-analysis involving over 4500 patients showing that chemotherapy reduces the risk of death in NSCLC by 10–20% [2]. This risk is clearly real for stage II and III NSCLC. For stage IB, which was studied in the CALGB study, the jury is still out, since only 1300 people in the meta-analysis had stage IB, so the overall power is still low.

Underpowered studies are a problem for many reasons. First, they can give misleading conclusions, which can hurt individuals and misdirect future research. Second, the people who volunteered for the study did so with the understanding that they were helping other people with their disease. We owe it to them to make sure their contribution was useful. (To be clear, negative studies are useful when we can stop or avoid doing things that are not helpful and when we can get other information about the disease from the study to guide future research. False-negative studies are less useful, however). Finally, low power is something to be thought about not only in terms of the conclusions of an individual study but also societal resources. The 2012 meta-analysis for postoperative chemotherapy in early-stage breast cancer included over 44,000 people in over 50 trials. We'll see in the next chapter about a very large trial in metastatic pancreatic cancer. One can legitimately ask why a trial in NSCLC, the most common cancer in the US, could not get enough power to answer the question about whether chemotherapy can increase the cure rate.

References

1. Strauss GM, et al. Adjuvant paclitaxel plus carboplatin compared with observation in stage IB non-small-cell lung cancer: CALGB 9633 with the Cancer and Leukemia Group B, Radiation Therapy Oncology Group, and North Central Cancer Treatment Group Study Groups. J Clin Oncol. 2008;26(31):5043–51.
2. Pignon JP, et al. Lung adjuvant cisplatin evaluation: a pooled analysis by the LACE Collaborative Group. J Clin Oncol. 2008;26(21):3552–9.

Overpowering

17

Some people argue that there is no such thing as a study that is too large, except for the money spent. More subjects mean more power, and more power can only be good. As the saying goes, if a little is good, then a lot must be better. However, like so many things in life, like alcohol, sugar, and chemotherapy, a lot of power in a study is not always good.

The issue is that the sample size of a study comparing two groups affects three things: the false-positive rate, the false-negative rate, and the detectable effect size in concert. The false-positive rate, called alpha, is controlled by the analysis and is the threshold at which a p-value will be considered significant. By convention, the false-positive rate is usually set at 0.05, or 5%. The false-negative rate, called beta, is the inverse of power, such that the power is 100% minus the false-negative rate. If the false-negative rate is 20% (or 0.2), the power is 80% (or 0.8). If the false-negative rate is 10%, the power is 90%. The detectable effect size is the difference between the groups that could be seen in the study. The units of effect size depend on what is being studied. For survival analyses, for example, effect sizes may be expressed as hazard ratios or as a difference between median survivals or as a difference between survival at a particular time.

Because the false-positive rate is fixed in the analysis, the sample size ends up determining the relationship between the power and the detectable effect size. Although in papers we write sentences like "with 450 people the study had an 80% power to detect a difference in median survival of 3 months," there is actually not one power and one detectable effect size of a study. For a fixed alpha (false-positive rate) and sample size, each power corresponds to a detectable effect size. So, if there is an 80% power to detect a difference in median survival of 3 months (meaning if the true difference is 3 months the study has an 80% chance of having a p-value at the end of less than 0.05), there may be a 90% power to detect a difference of 5 months (meaning if the true difference in survival is 5 months the study has a 90% chance of having a p-value at the end of less than 0.05), and a 50% power to detect a difference of 1 month (meaning that if the true difference in survival is 1 month the study has a 50% chance of having a positive p-value at the end).

© The Author(s), under exclusive license to Springer Nature Switzerland AG 2023
A. L. Cohen, *Problems and Pitfalls in Medical Literature*,
https://doi.org/10.1007/978-3-031-40295-1_17

The problem with very large studies (other than being a waste of money and people) becomes apparent. When a study is very large, the power to detect small, meaningless differences increases. We, thus, run the risk of having positive studies that are clinically useless because the difference detected is so small.

One classic example of an overpowered study was the cooperative group study NCIC CTG PA.3, which was a phase III clinical trial in metastatic pancreatic cancer comparing the standard chemotherapy of gemcitabine with a combination of gemcitabine and erlotinib, which was an exciting new targeted drug at the time of the study [1]. A total of 569 people were enrolled and randomized equally to the two treatment arms and then followed until they died. The trial was designed with an 80% power to detect a hazard ratio of 0.75 between the groups with an alpha of 0.05. We talked about hazard ratios in the proportional hazard chapter, but to give an idea of what this means, consider that the median survival of metastatic pancreatic cancer treated with gemcitabine at that time was about 6 months. A hazard ratio of 0.75 would increase that to less than 8 months. Thus, as planned, they were hoping to make people live about 6 weeks longer, which would not exactly be a triumph of modern medicine. However, as discussed above, that means the chance of having a positive study if the true difference is shorter than 6 weeks was not low.

And that is exactly what happened. The study was a positive study with a p-value of 0.038 and a hazard ratio of 0.82, which makes for a nice soundbite about people living almost 20% longer and being the first study to show a survival improvement with a targeted drug in pancreatic cancer. However, the actual numbers are less impressive. The median survival in the gemcitabine group was 5.91 months. The median survival in the combination group was 6.24 months. The curves were fairly parallel with no change in separation over time, so on average people lived 0.33 months longer with combination treatment (Fig. 17.1). For a 30-day month, that means that erlotinib made people live 10 days longer. By 18 months the same proportion of people were alive in each group, which was less than 5%. How much would you pay to live 10 days longer? For me, the answer is not much if anything. Although this study led to the inclusion of erlotinib on guidelines and pathways, FDA approval of erlotinib for use in metastatic pancreatic cancer, and further studies of this and similar drugs, all of which have been negative, it has been generally considered by the medical community as an example of a drug where the benefits do not outweigh toxicity in this population.

To avoid problems with an overpowered trial, study planners must think critically not just about how much money they have but also what a clinically meaningful difference in outcomes (effect size) is. Determining the clinically meaningful difference to target is not about statistics or resources. It is about knowing the disease and the priorities of the population affected by the disease. In some diseases and to some populations a 2-month improvement in survival may be meaningful while for others, they would only be interested in living years longer. Several resources can be used to determine an appropriate effect size to target. Some national organizations have put forth proposed targets for clinical trial goals. For example, ASCO, the American Society of Clinical Oncology, in 2014 proposed that 3–4 months was the appropriate goal to shoot for in certain people with metastatic

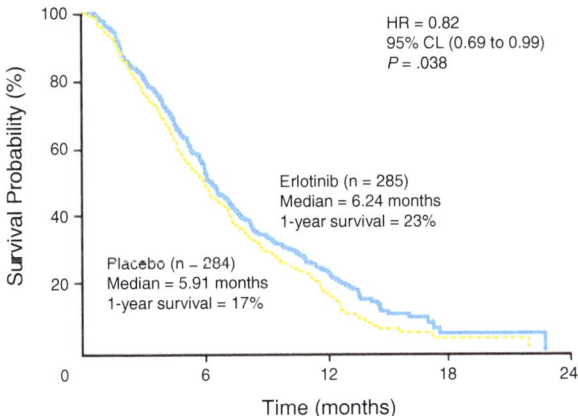

Fig. 17.1 Survival curves showing a statistically significant but clinically meaningless difference. (Reprinted with permission from Moore MJ, Goldstein D, Hamm J, Figer A, Hecht JR, Gallinger S, et al. Erlotinib plus gemcitabine compared with gemcitabine alone in patients with advanced pancreatic cancer: a phase III trial of the National Cancer Institute of Canada Clinical Trials Group. J Clin Oncol. 2007;25(15):1960 6)

pancreatic cancer but that in metastatic breast cancer, a 4–6 month improvement in survival should be the goal Patient advocates and patient representatives should also be an important part of such discussions because they represent the people actually affected by decisions about how large to make a trial.

Reference

1. Moore MJ, et al. Erlotinib plus gemcitabine compared with gemcitabine alone in patients with advanced pancreatic cancer: a phase III trial of the National Cancer Institute of Canada Clinical Trials Group. J Clin Oncol. 2007;25(15):1960–6.

Conclusion

I hope you have enjoyed this tour through the potential pitfalls in medical studies and clinical trials. In many ways, they overlap and boil down to a few themes. First, beware of studies that are too big or too small, particularly the small ones, which carry multiple risks for random results. Second, know what questions are being asked and whether they were asked before or after the study started. Third, just because something can be calculated doesn't mean it should be. Lastly, know a few common biases that you can watch for and see if they were adjusted by.

Many of the biases and pitfalls overlap. In the end, it doesn't matter whether a particular instance is called confounding by indication or selection bias. What matters is recognizing the particular issue and whether it is mitigated or not.

I like to stay in practice by looking at headlines and article titles and thinking about what biases may be present. You can try it on some of these and keep it in mind when reading journals or the newspaper:

From *the New York Times*—"These 90-year-old Runners Have Some Advice for You: You've got to Keep Moving."

Selection bias and immortal time bias

From *ASCO News*—"Patients with Advanced NSCLC Treated with Nivolumab May Live Longer when they Continue Treatment Instead of Stopping After a year."

Confounding by severity and immortal time bias

From *HealthDay*—"Reduced melanoma thickness is observed for those who receive screening for skin cancer."

Length time bias

From *MedPage Today*—"Patients whose lung cancer was detected by LDCT screening had a significantly lower 3-year incidence of brain metastases."

Length time bias and lead time bias

From *Medscape*—"Women with a breast cancer diagnosis who recalled eating nuts were not here found to have significantly better disease free survival over a 10-year study period compared with those who said they had not eaten nuts."

Recall bias, multiple comparisons, selection bias, confounding

A. L. Cohen, *Problems and Pitfalls in Medical Literature*, https://doi.org/10.1007/978-3-031-40295-1

From *Oncology Nurse Advisor*—"A therapeutic drug monitoring approach to treatment with dasatinib was shown to be associated with reduced rates of pleural effusion."

Hawthorne effect, confounding by indication

Index